Ask Me
About
My Uterus

Ask Me About My Uterus

A QUEST TO MAKE DOCTORS BELIEVE IN WOMEN'S PAIN

Abby Norman

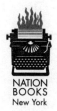

NATION
BOOKS
New York

Nation Books
116 East 16th Street, 8th Floor New York, NY 10003
www.publicaffairsbooks.com/nation-books
@NationBooks
Printed in the United States of America

First Edition: March 2018

Published by Nation Books, an imprint of Perseus Books, LLC, a subsidiary of Hachette Book Group, Inc.

Nation Books is a co-publishing venture of the Nation Institute and Perseus Books.

The Hachette Speakers Bureau provides a wide range of authors for speaking events. To find out more, go to www.hachettespeakersbureau.com or call (866) 376-6591.

The publisher is not responsible for websites (or their content) that are not owned by the publisher.

Print book interior design by Amy Quinn.

The Library of Congress has cataloged the hardcover edition as follows:

Names: Norman, Abby, author.
Title: Ask me about my uterus : a quest to make doctors believe in women's pain / Abby Norman.
Description: First edition. I New York : Nation Books, 2018. I Includes bibliographical references and index. I
Identifiers: LCCN 2017043712 (print) I LCCN 2017047259 (ebook) I ISBN 9781568585826 (ebook) I ISBN 9781568585819 (hardcover)
Subjects: LCSH: Norman, Abby—Health. I Endometriosis—Patients—Biography. I Endometriosis—Diagnosis. I Women—Health and hygiene. I BISAC: HEALTH & FITNESS / Women's Health. I BIOGRAPHY & AUTOBIOGRAPHY / Personal Memoirs.
I HEALTH & FITNESS / Pain Management.
Classification: LCC RG483.E53 (ebook) I LCC RG483.E53 N67 2018 (print) I DDC 618.1—dc23
LC record available at https://lccn.loc.gov/2017043712

ISBNs: 978-1-56858-581-9 (hardcover); 978-1-56858-582-6 (e-book)

LSC-C

10 9 8 7 6 5 4 3 2 1

To Hillary (the best thing that ever happened to me)
and Jax (the best thing that ever happened to her).

CONTENTS

Author's Note . . . .*xi*

Prologue 1
Chapter 1 5
Chapter 2 19
Chapter 3 57
Chapter 4 97
Chapter 5 111
Chapter 6 131
Chapter 7 187
Chapter 8 217
Chapter 9 235
Epilogue 257

Acknowledgments *261*
Notes. *267*

Each patient carries his own doctor inside him.

—Norman Cousins, *Anatomy of an Illness*

AUTHOR'S NOTE

IT IS MY SINCEREST HOPE that some of what is in this book will no longer be applicable by the time it's in your hands. Though a work becoming outdated may be embarrassing to some authors, as someone who is ill, I would be overjoyed if, in the time it took for this book to be published, science and society will have found answers to some of the questions I grapple with in these pages.

This book could never be fully comprehensive, and the research I've chosen to include represents only a fraction of what I encountered as a young patient parsing through it. Despite my determination, much to my dismay, I could never know all that there was to know, and as a reader I hope you will view all that I have written with a keen and critical eye. It was very important to me that I produce a portable book, so my ambition was not to provide a comprehensive history or review of the literature pertaining to women, illness, and pain. Rather, it was to provide some starting points from which you might seek to ask further questions and discover better answers.

Although this book includes research and interviews, I have framed the conversation around my own experience—not because I believe I can speak for anyone else, but because it seemed important to use the platform I have been given to call out the injustices I have observed (and in some cases experienced firsthand).

When debating the title for this book, I worried that it would be viewed as exclusionary to those who identify with the struggles portrayed but who do not have a uterus. I am firm in my conviction that endometriosis is not a uterine-dependent disease—as firm as I am in my conviction that not all women have a uterus and not all those who have a uterus identify as a woman. I do identify as a woman, and in telling this story I had to acknowledge what that identity meant in my journey. In the grander scheme of things, however, it should be noted that by no means is my having a uterus (for the time being, anyway) a requirement for my female identity, any more than it would be for anyone else.

I do not wish to become a poster girl, or "the voice of" anything depicted in this book: my experience is just one of many, and it is also one that benefited from the privilege of being a white woman. Where I have acknowledged how race and gender identity factor into my experiences in the broader sense, I have done so with the knowledge that there are others who could tell their own stories. We need to actively seek them out and listen to them.

Of course, there could never be one voice, or one story, that is wholly representative of the issues that are discussed in this book. But the voices of those who need to tell their stories have long been silenced. I offer up my own account to join what I hope will become many voices demonstrating the complexity of these issues, of ourselves, and of the fierce will of the human spirit.

In the same way that this book could never address all the research, it could not address every single event or person or conversation. I have, for the purpose of narrative and consideration for people involved in my story, obscured people's identities, changed their names, and occasionally altered times and places (including those of all my doctors). The dialogue included in this book most often came directly from journal entries written promptly after the events described, though a few of the more recent ones are re-created from my memory. Interviews were recorded, transcribed, and condensed for inclusion, or, in some cases, conducted via online exchanges.

Finally, it should be noted that any and all references to *The X-Files* or any other popular cultural phenomenon are not nearly as gratuitous as they may at first appear.

Abby Norman
June 2017

PROLOGUE

IT ALL STARTED WHEN I took what I now consider to be the worst shower of my life.

I was a sophomore at Sarah Lawrence College, living with my roommate Rebecca in a small house on campus; it was entirely unremarkable, except for the giant katydid that had spent weeks living above our bedroom door.

Rebecca had groaned in her sleep when my alarm went off, burying her head under her pillow. This was always our first exchange in the morning, even if she wasn't conscious for it. We'd met the first week of freshman year and our sense of humor and taste for hummus and good coffee had made us fast friends. I was a bit frantic by nature, always early, generally a bit wary of life. Rebecca was more laid back, except where social justice was concerned—in that domain, she was all action and advocacy, which inspired me from the outset. In general, she engaged in age-appropriate life experiences with gusto, while I was more hesitant. She was also the antithesis of a "morning person."

I had rolled out of bed on that otherwise unremarkable morning having had no premonitions of terror in my sleep. I grabbed my

1

towel and shower caddy, opened the door, and glanced at that freak-
ish katydid as I padded down the hall to the bathroom. I remember
looking out the small window that faced campus as I undressed, the
hour early enough that the world was quiet and still. The leaves had
begun to change, but fall in New York could not rival the fire trees of
where I had grown up in Maine. I'm from what you might call sturdy
New England stock, and I had all but shed the lingering jowliness
of a Maine accent. I wasn't ashamed of where I'd come from—quite
the contrary. I carried myself with what I'm sure was a rather pronounced affectation of New England pragmatism that bordered on
elitism, despite the fact that I'd grown up in a seaport—about as un-
pretentious as you can get.

Although I had no intention of living in Maine ever again—
having arrived in New York full-stop at eighteen, as many people
do—I did sometimes miss its breathtaking natural beauty. New York
City was stunning, too, but in a very different way. I'd never been
in the shadows of such tall buildings before, and the pulse of the
city thrummed in me long after I'd boarded the Metro-North back
to Bronxville. But I'd grown up a stone's throw from the ocean, in a
town whose maritime history was inextricably linked with my own.
We were all the descendants of sea captains, and the seashore was
often the only place I'd felt safe and protected as a child. I would lie
down in the wet sand, cross my arms over my chest, and wait for the
waves to come in and break against me. As they receded, they would
pull me into a tepid embrace that was warmer than anything I'd received from the human beings in my life.

Miles and years and states away, I stuck my hand in the shower,
letting the warm water wake up my fingers. Down the hall, bongo
drums began to thump, filling me with a sense of prescient nostalgia.
As I stepped into the tub and pulled the curtain closed, I wondered,
half asleep, if I was in the process of solidifying a memory.

That's when it happened, and it was as sudden as a thunderclap.
A stabbing pain in my middle, as though I were on the receiving end
of an unseen assailant's invisible knife.

I was immediately jolted awake, eyes wide and stinging. I pressed
a hand against my side, trying to determine exactly where it hurt. It
felt like it was everywhere and nowhere all at once. It was almost as

though something had snapped deep inside me. I had never experienced anything like it. I stood very still and closed my eyes, trying to drown out the bongo drums long enough to listen to my body.

The pain became more of an ache, which spread through my lower belly and pelvis, then snaked around my flank toward my back. I began to grow nauseated and dizzy. I fumbled to turn off the shower, tripping as I tried to step over the lip of the tub. My legs were shaking so much I could barely walk. From the floor I held my breath, waiting for the room to right itself so I could stand. I retched as I crawled across the floor, finally managing to pull myself up to the sink.

I wiped the fogged-up mirror and cringed at my reflection: bloodless skin and dark, wide eyes. I recoiled at the haunting image of my mother staring back at me.

To say I hadn't thought of my mother in years would be a lie, but I had not seen her so vividly for quite some time. The last place I'd wanted to see her was in the mirror, the reflection of my own face.

CHAPTER 1

The merest schoolgirl, when she falls in love, has
Shakespeare or Keats to speak her mind for her;
but let a sufferer try to describe a pain in his
head to a doctor and language runs dry.

—Virginia Woolf, "On Being Ill"

IN THE 1940S, A GROUP of researchers at Cornell University were trying to come up with an objective method to use in measuring pain. They suggested that a person's pain threshold be measured in a unit they called the *dol*, which was short for *dolor*—Latin for "pain." Once they had a name, they had to figure out what a *dol* actually was. The only way to do this was to design experiments that intentionally inflicted various types of pain onto human subjects, then scale them accordingly. So that's exactly what they did: they came up with over a hundred different experiments using various pain-inflicting stimuli. As they reached the upper limits of pain, however, they were confronted with a very obvious problem. To understand pain at that level, they'd have to truly injure a subject, and the margin of error for something like that would have no doubt been very small. What they needed was a highly painful experience that wasn't going to maim or kill anybody, and that they could easily observe. And that's how researchers from Cornell found themselves in the obstetric wing of New York Hospital burning the hands of laboring women.

The results of the study were published in 1949. It might seem like the study's authors would have had a lot of convincing to do when it came to recruiting women to take part, but, as they noted in their introduction, it actually wasn't that hard. The majority of the women volunteered because they were curious about the work. Many of them were either married to doctors or had been nurses, and they understood the challenge that pain presented to the field of medicine. They were, however, a little dubious about the proposed method. "Most of the patients commented upon the fact that the sensation from the uterus would be different in quality, duration and locale, and, therefore, expressed some doubt as to the possibility of equating the two sensations in terms of intensity," the authors wrote, though they noted that those concerns were not "borne out by experience," and that the majority of the women cooperated in describing their pain without issue.

The experiment went like this: as the thirteen women in the study labored, in between contractions the researchers would burn one of their hands with a thermal device the researchers had calibrated to deliver varying levels of intensity. The researchers had set the value of a dol as "approximately one-tenth the intensity of the maximal pain," which they were hoping the experiment would help them establish. What they really needed was for the women to be able to compare not just the intensity of the two types of pain, but their qualities. Of course, as the labor progressed, the women were understandably less communicative than at the outset, and so the researchers made inferences about their pain experience by noting their behaviors, "such as—crying, complaining, sweating and degree of alertness and cooperation." Not surprisingly (to women, anyway), the pain experienced by at least one of the women achieved the maximum value for the dol pain-measurement scale—a 10.5, what the researchers called "the most intense pain which can be experienced."

These experiments in dolorimetry provided a lot of fascinating data about pain, and it scientifically confirmed what women had known for millennia: that childbirth can push beyond the perceived limits of the human pain threshold. It did not, however, provide medicine with the kind of objective measurement it needed in terms of pain assessment. As compelling as the dol studies were, they still relied on the patient's willingness and ability to report their pain, which was inherently subjective.

Of the research that was done to try to establish a truly objective measure of pain throughout the twenty-first century, what most people are probably familiar with is the 0–10 pain scale. The concept seems straightforward enough: you ask patients where their pain is on a scale of 0–10. Zero is no pain, and 10 is the worst pain they can imagine. Presumably, when patients report something somewhere in the middle, they're comparing their current pain to previous painful experiences. Women who have given birth might compare a present pain to that of childbirth: "Not as bad as late-stage labor." Or, if a patient has previously broken a bone, he or she might say, "Well, it's worse than the time I broke my leg."

Since we all have varying degrees of tolerance for pain, and have equally varied experiences with different types of pain, it makes the scale feel kind of meaningless—especially when you consider that the person trying to ascertain how much pain the patient is in has his or her own experiences with pain that are thrown into the mix, too. A doctor trying to figure out how much pain a patient is in, when she says it's "worse than a broken leg," but "not as bad as childbirth," is still only going to be able to guess what that means based on his or her own experience—and perceptions—of pain.

This is true for any human being who witnesses another human being's pain. When I was in the fourth grade, my best friend, Hillary, went to lift the grate off the top of a fire pit in her backyard, not realizing it retained the heat of the smoldering coals beneath, and suffered severe burns to both of her hands, which required, to my ten-year-old eyes, an impressive amount of bandaging. I remember helping her write her classwork, turning the pages of her books in school, and watching as she winced whenever any pressure, even the lightest playground breeze, touched the raw, pink skin.

I knew she was in pain, but I couldn't know exactly how she felt. I had experienced a few childhood injuries that were pretty bad—the screaming, crying, bleeding kind—and I imagined it probably felt like that. But I couldn't know for sure what it felt like to be in her body, and I found that deeply disconcerting. She was my best friend, and I wanted to take her pain away. But how could I, when I didn't understand it?

⸻❧⸻

BY LOOKING BACK THROUGH EMAILS, social media posts, and medical records, I can piece together what happened after I stepped out of my ill-fated shower that autumn day. I don't remember exactly how I got from the bathroom back to the bedroom I shared with Rebecca. I don't remember if the bongo drums were still beating beneath the loud swell of my heartbeat in my ears. I don't remember whether the katydid flinched when I pushed my way back into the room, collapsing onto the bed. Nor do I remember how long I stayed there, curled up in the fetal position, before Rebecca woke up, shocked to find me there and not in class.

I do know that I didn't miss an entire day, because that afternoon I took a picture of myself in class to send to Hillary back home. We'd been best friends since preschool, twenty-some years of sisterhood that was wildly envied by most of the people who knew us. Since we were now living several states apart, we often sent daily photos, texts, or videos to one another, and at the very least were always connected through whatever metaphysical sisterly magic had bonded us as little girls.

In the photograph, I have my hair up in a messy bun. I'm wearing a big sweater and looking away from the camera, and I seem exhausted and miserable. The image triggers the next cascade of memories for me: I was in my biology lecture, which I hadn't wanted to miss, but I couldn't concentrate. I don't think I managed to take any notes, and as soon as it ended, I limped back across campus and went back to bed, having accomplished nothing aside from wearing myself out. The pain had reduced itself to a dull, almost undulating ache, a perfect storm ascending inside of me.

I felt feverish, nauseated, and like I couldn't keep my eyes open. I slept for the rest of the day and the better part of the next. I found it impossible to get comfortable: sitting up, lying down, fetal position, everything felt miserable. It felt like there was something inside of my body that was going to "pop" if I lay on my side or twisted my torso. I didn't eat for days; it became hard to sleep. By the time my weekend shift at my work-study job rolled around, almost a week later, I had started to accept that something was seriously wrong. I remember showing up and putting the coffee on—and collapsing. For the first time in years, I cried. Inexhaustibly, snottily, hard. I told Rebecca I was sick and needed to go to the hospital, and her dark eyes regarded me with bewilderment. I don't think I'd let on, until that moment, how bad I truly felt. Not even to myself.

If you're wondering why I had waited about a week before going to the hospital, despite being quite obviously ill, the answer is a complicated one. There was the practical concern about cost, because I didn't have decent health insurance. Many of my peers had benefited from the freshly minted Affordable Care Act, which allowed them to stay on their parents' health insurance plans until they were twenty-six. I had forfeited all that upon my emancipation at age sixteen, and I was extremely concerned about how I would pay for the cost of any care I received, not to mention any medications I might be prescribed. God forbid that I'd have to figure out how to pay for a hospital admission.

Another element of my reluctance to seek help was deeply rooted in my personal psychology, part of a complex belief system I hadn't yet been able to shed. As a little girl, whenever I would get sick with some routine childhood illness, my mother implored me to "talk myself out of it." She was exhausted from her own illness and its antecedent psychological torture, and she didn't have the energy to take care of a sick kid.

She was particularly harsh and unfeeling toward me if I had a stomach upset of some kind. I can only assume that my throwing up was a highly triggering event for her, given her illness. If I approached her for comfort in those long, seemingly endless dark nights of my childhood ailments, she rejected me. I took her revulsion personally, as I think any child would, and vowed never to get sick again. I began to use all my mental fortitude to "talk myself out of it" whenever I took ill, so that life could resume as per usual—for Mum and me both. There were occasions, of course, when I couldn't use mind over matter. When I inevitably did throw up, or have a fever, or get strep throat for the umpteenth time in a given year, I internalized those instances as personal failings.

Yet another contributing factor was that the first time I had trusted a doctor, she had let me down. I know now that there are complexities to reporting suspected child abuse. I know that the suspicion must be high, that there must be proof. Given that I was hardly out of elementary school at the time, all I knew was that I was scared and hungry—and that white coats meant someone knew a hell of a lot and had power to make you better.

At some point as a child I'd developed an elevator pitch of my situation, trying to be ready for the oft-wished-for but never manifested opportunity when I would be alone with an adult who might be able to help me. I've never been a particularly succinct individual, though, so while my pitch was well articulated in my head, it never seemed to form as a cohesive statement. Instead it just sounded like a series of sighs and mumbles, along with the occasional throaty hack of nervous laughter.

The pediatrician asked my mother to leave the room when I was, if my memory serves, there for a routine immunization. I couldn't have been more than ten or eleven. My mouth went dry and my heartbeat ached in my ears. I don't know if I was old enough yet to have the words "Don't fuck it up" in my lexicon, but I very much had the feeling. As predicted, I didn't stay cool, and it all came tumbling, dripping, cascading out of me. A truth purge.

The doctor's wide-eyed look, which I construed as disbelief, was quickly replaced by a slap of fear. She wasn't looking at me agog because of what I'd told her, but because my mother (who had been listening outside the door) had burst into the room. She seethed as she yanked me from the exam table and dragged me out into the hallway. The pediatrician followed us into the hall, but no farther, and I craned my neck to look back. I implored her with my eyes to do something. But she didn't. She only stared at me with an expression of gaunt helplessness.

My mother flung me into the car, and I awaited sentencing for my transgression with the sincere hope that it would be something akin to her driving the car off the bridge into the frigid water below, killing us both. But she kept her anger in her jaw, clenched like a bear trap, until she could get home to release it.

I swallowed mine.

A DECADE OR SO LATER, before any doctor doubted my pain, I doubted it myself, because that's what my mother had taught me to do. I was nineteen years old and didn't want to be sick. It wasn't even a question of want—I simply *couldn't* be sick. I had to go to class. I was on a massive scholarship that was contingent on my academic success. I had friends to see, dances to do, a spectacular city within reach. I had so much life to live, and for the first time ever I was completely free of all that had hurt me and stolen my joy. That morning in the bathroom, as pain ripped through me like a bullet and I saw my mother's face on my own, I tried harder than ever to talk myself out of being sick.

By the time I ended up in the hospital, I was inconsolable. Did I not want to be at Sarah Lawrence badly enough? Was I really so weak-willed and pathetic that I was getting worked up over a silly, stupid little ailment? I was becoming delirious from not eating, and I hadn't been drinking much of anything, either. The pain in my belly had become all-consuming.

I sat slumped in a chair in the intake room. At first the nurse in triage seemed doubtful of my pain, because I was so subdued from all the crying that I just stared, glassy-eyed, at the wall. As she took my blood pressure, she seemed dubious. I had reported that the reason for my visit was a frightening amount of abdominal pain, and I guess she expected me to be screaming and rolling around on the floor. But the pain had exhausted me to the point of surrender. When I was taken back to a curtained cubicle, I dragged my book bag with me. Despite the fact that I could hardly keep my eyes open and would occasionally burst into tears, I was consumed by the reality that the following week I had a test to pass in my Russian class. Russian, as it turned out, was a difficult language to learn. Every second of studying counted, and since I'd been sick all week, I'd missed class as well as my tutoring session. I frantically tried to conjugate verbs, partially out of fear, but also as a method of distraction.

Aside from that morning, when I'd woken up and taken the notably apocalyptic shower, the only other time I'd experienced something that required me to go to the hospital in Bronxville had occurred about six months earlier, when a dance injury had ended in an ankle splint. That visit had been uneventful, relatively speaking.

It wasn't until I landed there in a weepy haze of terror that I actually took stock of the place. The emergency room was considerably more attractive than it needed to be. I was used to small-town hospitals that were a little on the dingy side and devoid of aesthetic frills.

Though it was a rather handsome hospital, once I got into the nurse's station to have my vitals taken, I was no longer paying attention to the decor. That was when they first asked me to rate my pain on a scale of 1–10. It was hardly my first encounter with the traditional pain scale, but something about that moment—and the many that would follow in the next five years—struck me as being somehow illogical.

Considering how sick I was, it wasn't the time to get hung up on semantics, yet I was—to the point of being almost indignant. It wasn't the nurse's fault; nor would it be the fault of the doctor who would ask me again a few hours later. And yet I was right to question the efficacy of a numerical pain scale that attempted to quantify an entirely subjective experience.

Doctors in emergency rooms don't have much investment in a patient's well-being. First of all, they don't have the time. Second, they have to maintain some professional detachment, or else they wouldn't make it through a single shift. The pain scale doesn't call on them to empathize with a patient, by attempting to understand their experience of pain, and supposedly, that makes it a good clinical tool. But even if it's a good tool for clinicians, it's not a good tool for patients.

The pain scale has many limitations. It's only concerned with the intensity of the pain, not the duration, for example, and it doesn't leave room for descriptions that provide essential information, such as "sharp," "dull," or "stabbing." These adjectives, though not reflected by the 1–10 labels, can actually be very helpful in creating a diagnostic portrait, because certain types of injury or infection can inflict certain types of pain.

In June 2005, *Harper's* ran a beautiful piece about the pain scale exploring its similarities to wind: "Wind, like pain, is difficult to capture," wrote the author, Eula Biss. "The poor windsock is always striving, and always falling short." Biss then eloquently explained that sailors eventually came up with a system to describe wind that consisted not just of a standardized numerical scale, but also names and categories for wind according to how it felt. It's called the Beaufort scale: "A force 2 wind on the Beaufort scale, for example, is a 'Light Breeze' moving between four and seven miles per hour," Biss wrote. "On land, it is specified as 'wind felt on face; leaves rustle; ordinary vanes moved by wind.'"

How would we describe a 2 on the pain scale? The twinge of a mosquito bite? An itch you mistakenly scratched with a too-sharp fingernail? Describing a subtle pain is generally more difficult than describing an all-consuming one. On the other end of that spectrum is the 10: the worst pain you can imagine.

The problem has always intrigued me, because I like to think I'm a fairly creative person. I'm sure I could imagine some pretty extreme situations in which I would feel immense pain. I have questions, though: Is a 10 meant to be a pain that would kill me? If that's the case, then how do you really measure the difference between a 9 and a 10? Are we physiologically capable of surviving a sustained 6 for a longer time than we could endure a brief 8?

There is another commonly used scale. It has cartoon faces wearing expressions that range from Kurt Vonnegut's "Everything is beautiful and nothing hurts!" to Leslie Knope's "Everything hurts and I'm dying." It was designed for children, and yet it's in about every doctor's office I've ever been in. None of which, over the past five years, have been pediatrician's offices.

But though it might be simpler, it's not necessarily any better than the numerical scale, at least in part because it confuses its intended audience: children are arguably even less able to separate physical from emotional pain than adults. In her *Harper's* piece, Biss explains that if you show the cartoon-face scale to a child who is scared, but not in pain, the child may still identify with the crying-pain face— the child misses the subtlety of the questions being asked.

But it's not only children who conflate physical and emotional pain. When I stared at that pain scale in the triage room, crying and scared myself, I certainly didn't identify with the faces that were just like "meh" about their pain. I was in pain, I was scared, and I was crying. Those three simultaneous realities didn't necessarily feel independent of each other.

Maybe kids have the right idea, though: If my pain is enough to make me afraid, shouldn't that stand to bump it up from, say, an *I'm-coping-okay* 4 to an *I'm-really-not-functioning* 5?

Later, writhing on a scratchy gurney, I perseverated on my answers to the pain-scale question because the nurse had seemed suspicious of me. Had I failed the test? Given the wrong answer? Should I have rounded down? Was my mother right to instill in me a tendency to play down my pain so that I wouldn't inconvenience other people? Was that what the nurses and doctors expected me to do? Was that what I had expected myself to do?

It felt strange to consider, as I lay there gray-faced looking up at a slightly less gray ceiling, that I should have lied. Yet I felt guilty, too, because the more I thought about it, the more I second-guessed my interpretation of a 6. My mind spun, trying to reason out how I'd arrived at an answer. The pain was bad enough that I couldn't ignore it, which made it definitely higher than a 4 or 5. It had been more painful a week ago, back when it had started—but then again, maybe I'd just grown accustomed to it. I couldn't tell.

What did the nurse think a 6 was? What would the doctor think that a 6 should be? Tears of frustration came. What was the point of this pain scale if they weren't going to believe me anyway?

By the time the doctor came in to examine me, I was even more exhausted than when I'd arrived. I was aware that I was still crying, and worried that while crying I couldn't possibly present my situation rationally. The doctor seemed completely unsurprised by my distress. I was a Sarah Lawrence girl—historically what you might call "bright and wound tight." He assumed that my issue was of a sexual nature, and it was only this assumption that managed to rouse me from my stupor.

Little did he know at that point that it couldn't possibly have had anything whatsoever to do with sex, because I was a virgin—a fact that I was somewhat embarrassed to admit. Still, I didn't want there to be any confusion, so I was firm in my assertion that he'd better come up with another diagnosis, because unless I was a modern-day biblical parable, there was no way I was pregnant. Nor was my body consumed by syphilis or any other sexually transmitted disease.

I'll admit that at nineteen, I didn't know much about sex, but there was one thing I did know: I wasn't having any.

He also seemed uncomfortable, which made me feel worse. I was suddenly flooded by memories of being warned not to be "difficult" as a child. I stopped talking after several futile attempts to explain, deciding maybe it would be easier if I didn't say anything at all. I was discharged without so much as a CT scan, prescribed a hefty dose of antibiotics, and encouraged to drink my weight in cranberry juice.

I spent the following week in bed, alternately crying and dry-heaving. I missed all of my classes (including the one where my fellow students took that Russian test). Instead, I made my way through Barbra Streisand's entire filmography.

By the time the weekend came, having not had anything to eat but saltines and cranberry juice, I went to the hospital a second time. My pain remained unchanged, and the antibiotics had done little, aside from giving me diarrhea (which seemed entirely unfair, given how weak I had been to begin with). I saw a different doctor the second time around. He, unlike the doctor before him, didn't balk at my tears, which were now a constant undercurrent rather than an occasional punctuation in the conversation. I'd started crying on Wednesday or so, and here it was Saturday and I hadn't stopped.

"When did you realize it was this bad?" the doctor asked me, his eyes kind but also looking back and forth rapidly between me and Rebecca, who had come along. I think she was as horrified by the scene as he was, if not more so.

"All I've done for a week is watch Barbra Streisand movies," I sobbed, not knowing what else to say. It was the truth, after all. I hadn't slept or eaten or gone to class—I'd been curled up in my bed with a pillow between my knees, watching *The Mirror Has Two Faces*, and wishing for death.

"That is serious," the doctor said, making a note in his chart. Having looked at my medical records since, I assure you that he did not write down, "*Prince of Tides*-induced sobbing" under my problem list. He just noted that I was clearly very upset, Babs notwithstanding.

Finally, I had the gamut of imaging tests, plus another liter or two of IV fluids, and then I fell into an exhausted half-sleep. I was motionless beneath the covers, my eyes tightly closed, as though I were rehearsing for my own death, when I felt the doctor's presence in the room. He sat down at the edge of the gurney, near my feet. It reminded me of how sometimes when I was a child, my father used to come into my bedroom after I'd gone to bed, not to tuck me in, per se, but to sit at the foot of the bed for a few minutes. Sometimes I would hear him making his way down the hallway, and I'd try to position my feet so that he'd end up sitting on them. He wouldn't hug me, he wouldn't kiss me good night. But for a few seconds I would feel the weight of him sitting on my feet, and I'd know he was real.

Even if I hadn't been too exhausted to move, I wouldn't have been so brazen as to stick my feet under the butt of an ER doctor I'd only just met. I felt myself begin to whimper again, the vestiges of my week-long cry-fest. He explained, first, that he had a daughter my age, and since he'd ascertained that I was only in New York for college, he wondered aloud if it would help to call my family back home. I told him no, there wasn't anyone to call. I didn't have the energy to explain the entire story to him, so I spat out the words "emancipated minor" and let him interpret it however he wanted. He did tense up a bit, as though he expected me to morph into some kind of shank-carrying delinquent who was there to steal drugs and wreak havoc, like a character in an Emmy-winning episode of *ER*.

He went on to explain that he didn't know what the problem was, but that he thought I could have an ovarian cyst, something that was very much a college-age-girl-thing. As it stood, maybe he'd seen it on the scan, or maybe he hadn't. He was just an ER doctor, not a gynecologist, so he wanted me to follow up with one of the latter. Beyond that, he just shrugged.

Bright and wound tight, Sarah Lawrence girls were. That was the enduring reason, the medical consensus, for my strife. I'd chosen the school for its focus on writing, sure—but not so that I could become my generation's answer to Sylvia Plath, fatal neuroses included.

I don't remember getting back to my dorm from the hospital that second time. I don't remember anything at all until the middle of the following week, when I had to go to the dean's office to discuss "my future." I hadn't been to class for several days, though I kept insisting that I would "surely feel better tomorrow," and "wouldn't have to drop the class, no, of course not."

As I sat shaking in the office, all I heard was "medical leave of absence" and "go home." I swallowed, my mouth and throat so dry that I was afraid that if I spoke, my tongue would shatter like glass.

"This is my home," I offered, and it sounded pathetic, but it was the truth. I didn't have a home to go back to. I hadn't had one at all until I came to Sarah Lawrence. While the dean was understanding about my situation, her hands were tied. I was there on a full scholarship that was contingent on academic performance. I had to take a leave of absence to heal. Clearly I needed to go somewhere to rest and recuperate, to try to get to the bottom of what was making me sick. I'd have to figure out where to do that. Preferably within the next week.

The problem was, I had not lived at home with my parents for six years. At age twelve, I had moved in with my grandmother. I was legally emancipated at sixteen, and I'd lived in several places in the two years that had elapsed between that day and the day I'd left for New York. There were a number of people who "looked out for me," but that was quite different from taking me in, were I to show up on their doorstep sick and alone. The last address where I had received mail was at the home of a woman named Rose-Leigh, who had taught at my high school and was an accomplished scientist. We had spent many late-summer afternoons identifying flora at her kitchen table over tea. Rose-Leigh had lost her youngest child some years before, and as a result of that unfathomable loss she always looked, to me, how grief felt. Although she was remarkably kind to me, and truly brilliant, what I remember most about her is the gray, almost woolen heaviness of her spirit.

Weighing my options, or lack thereof, I plodded unsteadily across the street and up the walkway to the office of my beloved psychology professor, Elizabeth. Her expression softened as she listened to my attempt to explain that I was sick and no one knew why, but that I wanted to be at Sarah Lawrence more than anything. My home was here, my heart was here, and I didn't want all my work to go to waste. I would be back in the spring, I vowed (or implored) and blubbered on as though, if I just sat there in her office long enough, and talked and talked and talked and never stopped, I wouldn't have to leave after all.

"Pausing isn't stopping," she told me, her earnest parting wisdom. I said goodbye to all my professors, and every single one of them said they looked forward to seeing me back in the spring. I never saw any of them again.

CHAPTER 2

*I know you are only a tiny little girl, but there is
some kind of magic in you somewhere.*

—Roald Dahl, *Matilda*

IF WOMEN HAVE BECOME SYNONYMOUS with hysteria, malingering, and hypochondria in a clinical setting, then it has far less to do with the natural inclinations of women and behavior than it does with the history of medicine. The medicalization of female internal sensations, which began as early as the 1800s, paved the way for the struggles modern women face in having their symptoms taken seriously in a medical setting.

Even outside of the doctor's office and in social settings, women face a constant barrage of doubt that undermines their faith in their own internal experiences. They begin to question their reality. It's not as though it has always been just patriarchal male doctors squelching women in the exam room—though patriarchal male doctors still do that. Women themselves have often subscribed to the wandering uterus theory of hysteria, mostly because they have been powerless to question it.

The reported symptoms of many of the women documented in early case studies of hysteria, such as Sigmund Freud's patient Dora, and a patient of his colleague Josef Breuer's named Anna O., are eerily reminiscent of what some of the women I've talked to in the present day have said. It's a symptom profile that includes both pelvic pain and vague abdominal pain—the origin of which is further complicated by its somewhat amorphous nature. They report grinding fatigue, both physical and mental, that is extremely difficult to articulate and even to comprehend. To fathom that level of fatigue, particularly when it has become chronic, and therefore begins to seem normal, is not only challenging, but legitimately depressing.

When I happened upon Gilda Radner's memoir several years ago, in the midst of my own medical turmoil, I grew deeply concerned about her life. The *Saturday Night Live* alum—wife of Gene Wilder and a gifted comedienne in her own right—left a lasting impression on me. I had not realized that she had died of ovarian cancer; nor had I realized that she was only forty-two years old when she did. What troubled me even more were the passages of her book recounting those final years of her life. It was the 1980s, and she was at the height of her popularity.

"My ovaries became the center of my universe," Radner wrote in *It's Always Something*. It was an eerie statement, considering what happened later, but she was referring to her struggle with infertility, which took place long before the word "cancer" was ever uttered to her as a diagnosis for her ailments. She and Wilder spent years in the slog of medical procedures that any couple undergoing in vitro fertilization (IVF) treatments must endure: the ultrasounds, the laparoscopies, the coming-into-a-cup. In her memoir she described the sequence, and one can't help but feel incredibly worried by the image of Gene Wilder—with his big, sad eyes—trying to ejaculate into a cup next to a stack of *Playboy* magazines in some nondescript, sterile, closet-like hospital room at the University of California at Los Angeles. When the IVF didn't take, Radner elected to have her tubes opened surgically. It was a risky alternative, since this type of "microsurgical technology" was still relatively new in the mid-1980s.

The surgery didn't exactly cure her of her ovarian-focused universe: Radner was then tasked with determining exactly when she was ovulating, so that she might maximize her chances of conceiving. She went out and bought an at-home ovulation kit ("Where you are the scientist," she wrote), but didn't tell Wilder what she was up to, as he'd been more than a bit traumatized by the whole IVF experience.

She recalled the fervor of one morning when she couldn't get the cap off the test vial. Desperate, she raced into the bedroom, poked a still fast-asleep Wilder, and said, "Don't ask me any questions, just take the lid off this vial." He did, and he never asked her about it—having done so while still fast asleep.

How could she have known, at that moment, in the early years of her marriage to Wilder, that the focus on her ovaries would never let up? That the very organs she doted upon—hoping as she did to cherish them into submission, so that they might bend to her will and give her a baby—were plotting to take her life? That even if she'd had a baby, she would have been dead before the child started school?

Radner's story haunted me, not because she was some comedic legend whose life was cut short, or just because she'd died from cancer in her ovaries, but because she had died as a result of her doctors not believing her when she said she was unwell. In fact, one doctor told Wilder that Radner was "a very nervous, emotional girl. She's got to relax."

The only thing any doctor could identify in Radner's lab tests was Epstein-Barr virus, which causes mononucleosis. That wasn't altogether unusual, as many people have the antibodies for it. Her symptoms persisted, however, and worsened. She would be fine for, say, ten days, and then, "seemingly around my menstrual cycle," she wrote, "I would go into this severe fatigue and run a low grade fever, then I would be okay again." She went to her gynecologist, who assured her that nothing was wrong; it was just "mittelschmerz," the sensation some women feel at the time of ovulation. "Now I had Epstein-Barr virus and mittleschmerz," she wrote. "Fitting diseases for the Queen of Neurosis."

Radner referred to herself as neurotic, and maybe she was. But neurotics get cancer too. Over the next few months, the grinding fatigue continued, as well as a seemingly never-ending plague of stomach and bowel problems. Her doctor said she was probably taking too many vitamins, although she had been told to take them to counteract the grinding fatigue she was experiencing. She saw yet another doctor who thought her stomach problems were—surprise!—the result of anxiety and depression. Then she got a new symptom: aching, gnawing leg pain. It started in her upper thighs and spread into her already weak legs. Her doctor gave her a high dose of anti-inflammatory medication, which caused her to have terrible nausea and vomiting. Her doctor then gave her medication to reduce the acid in her stomach, so that she could take the anti-inflammatory medication. The leg pain worsened. Her doctors told her to take a Tylenol.

Ever determined to prove she was ill, even as she began to physically waste away, Radner saw a doctor in Boston—who gave her an antidepressant. When she didn't seem immediately placated, he asked her what she was so afraid of. "I am afraid that it is cancer," she told him. He told her to just keep having her blood drawn and to stay in touch with her doctor, "so that you can set your mind at ease."

She went home. She tried acupuncture. Holistic medicine. She took supplements. The pain in her legs kept her up at night. She bloated so severely that she really did look pregnant—which must have been such a fantastically cruel reminder that she had not been able to conceive.

Radner dutifully kept having blood drawn, and then, finally, on October 20, 1986—ten months of her insistence later—her doctor called. Her liver function, he said, was irregular. She asked him what that meant.

"It's probably nothing," he said, but he wanted her to come in anyway. It was Stage IV ovarian cancer.

"Gilda cried," Wilder recalled in an essay he wrote for *People*. "But then she turned to me and said, 'Thank God, finally someone believes me!'"

The "treatment" was a complete hysterectomy, which dashed any lingering hope for conceiving a child that she may have harbored. Then, intense chemotherapy and radiation, which made her so sick that those around her thought she would die—and she, at times, wanted to. The experience irrevocably changed her, a fact that became obvious, even on her good days.

"No one recognized me at all," she wrote. "I began to introduce myself as, 'I used to be Gilda Radner.' That was how it felt. I used to be her, but now I was someone else."

In the two years after she was diagnosed, while undergoing treatment, she also began working on the memoir, one that focused heavily on her experience. She knew even as she was still very much *in* her "weird life," as she called it, that her experiences might help someone else—even if it was too late to use the knowledge she'd gained for her own benefit. After Radner's death in 1989, Wilder continued her work, becoming an advocate for research and awareness up until his death in 2016.

"For weeks after Gilda died, I was shouting at the walls. I kept thinking to myself, 'This doesn't make sense,'" Wilder wrote in a guest article in *People* two years after her death. "The fact is, Gilda didn't have to die. But I was ignorant, Gilda was ignorant—the doctors were ignorant."

When I finished reading her memoir, I listened to the audiobook she had recorded of it just a week before her death. Her voice is at times alarmingly thready, almost hollow. I know she was still alive when she recorded it, but as I listened, I couldn't help but feel like she had already become a ghost. The exhaustion in her voice as she recalled her unceasing attempts to convince doctors that she was ill—and later, at their urging, to convince herself that she was not—echoed through me, resonating painfully.

As Radner wondered aloud in her memoir, what came first, the illness or the depression? Was being sick making her depressed, or was depression making her sick? How many of us have asked that same question, or ask it almost daily as we slog forward in time? It's the Ouroboros of pain from which we cannot escape, no matter how hard we try, unequivocally felt by us and questioned by everyone else—until we, too, are forced to doubt the veracity of our reality. I couldn't help but wonder as I pored over Radner's memoir what would have happened if it had been another body system afflicted. Radner had started smoking at the age of fourteen. What if she'd had lung cancer instead? Would she have been taken seriously the first time she reported symptoms? Would she have received a diagnosis sooner? Would the treatments available to her have been more curative, because more research and attention is paid to cancers like that?

If I, or any other woman whose gynecologic cancers or pathologies had gone undiagnosed, had just been sick in some other part of the body, in some other way, would it have been any different? Or would it not have mattered? Was the underlying preexisting condition being female? Does the congenital lack of a Y chromosome predispose a patient to worse outcomes regardless of what condition or disease they present with?

—※—

DURING THE 1600S, SEVERAL MALE physicians, such as John Sadler and William Harvey, asserted that the uterus was the seat of all ills in a woman—and that the organ itself was central to the body. Whatever it felt would influence everything else: the rest of her body followed suit. It was almost seen as a possession, of sorts, and often it was excised, removed in the hope that the woman's symptoms would disappear once her unruly womb was gone.

The womb itself has often been viewed as something of a live animal within the body cavity, a unique distinction that does not apply to other, lesser organs. A familiar notion in Central Europe was that the uterus was animalistic: the womb was sometimes referred to as a *muttern* (German for "toad"). The symbolism was based in the idea that the uterus was capable of "hopping around" inside a woman's body.

Hysteria was something of a catch-all diagnosis in its day. Symptoms ranged from the frustratingly vague to the impressively grotesque, and the uterus was almost always blamed for a hysteric woman's suffering. It was all supposedly explained by something called "reflex theory," which meant, essentially, that physical symptoms resulted from mental overexertion, excessive emotions, and the like.

It's no easier today to describe one's internal sensations and physical experience, but during the latter part of the twentieth century, the task was further complicated by a simple lack of understanding about how the central nervous system functioned.

It was also (and arguably still is) difficult for medical professionals to assess irritation versus inflammation. Irritation can be experienced by a patient and articulated, but it cannot be measured. Inflammation, on the other hand, is also often felt, but can be detected through bloodwork or examination of the affected tissues. John Burns, a Scottish physician in the 1800s, was one of the first to really study the two. He tried not to use the terms interchangeably, because he did not believe they were the same. The concept of "irritation" was a broad one, and could be used to legitimize almost anything a doctor encountered, whereas "inflammation" could be traced to some biophysical marker, something that could be felt and seen. "Irritation" could cloud over cases where inflammation was present, but only sporadically or on a cyclic schedule. This kind of thinking also furthered the widely held belief that people (women, in particular) could be "excitable," and thus, that their lives could be improved by trips to the seaside for a rest—or tidily hidden away in an asylum. Or an attic. If a woman was not actually sent out of the home, she may well have been made prisoner in her own house, her own bedroom, even—a la Charlotte Perkins Gilman's "The Yellow Wallpaper."

"Nervous disease" was a term more descriptive of a patient's personality than of a patient's actual, physical nervous system, especially when the patient was a woman. The hustle and bustle of modern life during the Industrial Revolution was thought to be so overwhelming, so overstimulating, that it was capable of causing a nervous collapse in those who were, perhaps, a little delicate. But at least since the 1700s, there had also been a distinct group of "nervous diseases" that were pathologic in nature, and weren't to be confused with the "nervous hysterias" of the era. These included visible lesions on the brain or spine (as in most cases of multiple sclerosis) as well as "functional" diseases, such as epilepsy, or other ailments that may have had organic causes that no one had yet discovered.

Unlike many of today's diseases, endometriosis included, by the mid-1800s hysteria had a pretty standard clinical presentation. If a patient exhibited a certain constellation of symptoms, she could quickly be diagnosed as a textbook hysteric. This development came in part thanks to the work of Jean-Martin Charcot, who believed that hysteria was a "real" malady, and not just something manufactured psychologically. It was he who began in earnest the search for the lesions that would qualify hysteria as an organic disease.

Charcot, to his credit, did for a time legitimize hysteria as an actual medical diagnosis: specifically, a neurological disorder. The creation of a clinical portrait is down to him: "In the hysterical attack," he wrote, "nothing is left to chance. To the contrary, everything unfolds according to the rules, which are always the same. They are valid for all countries, epochs, races—in short, universal."

By looking at brains postmortem, Charcot began to try to correlate the symptoms a patient had demonstrated with abnormalities in the brain. It was through this investigation that he discovered diseases such as amyotrophic lateral sclerosis, or ALS, today often called Lou Gehrig's disease. Hysteria, he believed, would be found in the brain and not the reproductive organs.

As anyone who has ever attempted to disprove the leading theory of anything will tell you, this did not go over well. He conceded that although the uterus may not be the seat of hysteria, the ovaries could be push-buttons for whatever neurological malfunction occurred. In an attempt to prove this theory, he devised a machine called an "ovary compressor," which was just as horrific as it sounds. Demonstrating on patients at the Salpêtrière, the mental asylum in Paris where he worked and did the bulk of his research, he would use the apparatus essentially to squash the ovaries of women in his care. They, of course, reacted in grandiose ways—in part because they were, no doubt, in great physical pain (which would not surprise anyone who has ever had a particularly rough pelvic exam). Some women, aware that hysterics were expected to behave according to a particular narrative, may have (consciously or unconsciously) felt the need to live up to (or even outdo) the behavioral precedent other patients had set.

Charcot's device was certainly encouraging the symptoms of hysteria to manifest—but it didn't explicitly prove that the ovaries were the impetus for them, or that there was even an organic neurological basis for the disease. Throughout his life—and evermore after his death—Charcot was frequently undermined by the rest of the medical establishment. His students took his research and reworked it after he died, claiming it as their own, and often used it to invalidate the theories he had presented.

Nor did patients remember Charcot very fondly: although he had come the closest of anyone, perhaps, to taking them "seriously," by suggesting that their symptoms and disease states were real, he hadn't hesitated to exploit the women in his care. They were an integral component of his famed, if not rather dramatic, series of lectures. Delivered from something of a pulpit adorned with footlights, his demonstrations, which were greatly admired by Freud, featured well-known patients at the Salpêtrière. They could go on for several hours, often drawing the attention of the public, who could come to gape as though they were taking in a circus side show.

Charcot's lectures and flagrant exposés may have been among the most entertaining of such demonstrations, but they weren't the only ones. Social mores of the era almost assured that the patient-physician dynamic be without boundary, and that meant women were vulnerable to exploitation—including sexual—regardless of whether they were "true hysterics" or not. It's not uncommon to read old patient charts in which sexual relations—consensual or not—between patients and physicians were noted simply as a matter of fact, implying that such a relationship was not thought to violate ethical standards. It helped that, during the mid-nineteenth century, sedation was becoming increasingly popular as a first line of treatment for women for just about anything—particularly ether, which was highly addictive. Women who were in a semiconscious state were obviously particularly vulnerable to physicians who wanted to exploit them.

The treatment of women by the medical establishment in the early twentieth century is further illuminated by the description of male hysteria, or *neurasthenia*. Neurasthenia was the kind of diagnosis a doctor might give a man he had known for years when he came in for a bad headache, before offering him a snifter of brandy. Hysteria was the diagnosis that same doctor would give a woman in the village who hadn't been able to walk for three weeks.

Male physicians were not the only ones carrying this narrative. The patriarchal structure of medicine informed how female physicians practiced, too—as much, if not more than, it did their male colleagues. At the expense, yet again, of female patients.

One physician of the era, Mary Putnam Jacobi of New York, bluntly compared male versus female hysteria, saying: "If this be a female, and notably selfish, the case is pronounced hysteria. If a man, or though a woman, amiable and unselfish, the case is called neurasthenia." Delving further into Jacobi's writing, one finds that she saw hysteria as a natural consequence of affluent white-lady boredom. Certainly in some cases this was true, just as it is today. There have always been, and there will always be, malingerers. But it's curious that throughout history, a woman in pain was presumed to be lying. Guilty until proven innocent, as it were.

Perhaps it was easier for a male doctor—who did not understand the intricacies of the female reproductive system, who could not fathom the feeling of a deep and unrelenting weight in one's pelvis, threatening to split the person in two—to call the woman a liar than admit he did not know what was wrong. That he did not know how to help her. Perhaps it was that women, who were so severely un-challenged, who were sequestered away with little or nothing in the way of intellectual opportunity, grew so bored that they devised a devilish scheme by which they could bring constant fascination into their lives, drawing attention to themselves. Perhaps they found iden-tity in illness. If so, I'm tempted to applaud them for their creativity, but also find myself angry at their short-sightedness—at what Jacobi called selfishness.

It was more than likely a combination of these and other psy-chosocial, cultural factors that created the essence of hysteria, from which not even the most modern of modern women have completely broken free. It lives in all of us, a little cough that makes us question our perceptions of ourselves, the innermost truth of our bodies, our very minds.

We've all done it. We've all gone to work with a fever and said, "It's nothing, just a cold," when we knew deep down we had the flu. We've rationalized having "food poisoning" for weeks as the real cul-prit digs its heels deeper into our guts. We've fainted, vomited, bled, laughed, screamed, and cried—and said, "I'm sorry, I don't know what came over me," when we know damn well, deep down, exactly what came over us: a wave of nausea, crushing fatigue, disorienting dizziness. If only we'd listen.

If only someone on the outside knew the language we speak in-side ourselves to keep our pain a secret, to silence our suffering, to find one hundred reasons why we're fine instead of the one reason that we're sick.

⸺⁂⸺

WHEN I WAS SEVENTEEN, ONE morning I noticed that I was having a hard time getting my feet to firmly hit the stairs. I grabbed the bannis-ter and laughed it off, thinking I must either not quite be awake or had slept weird and irritated a nerve in my leg. I brushed it off and carried on with my day assuming it would resolve. But the next morning, the same thing happened. Then I started having difficulty using the stairs at school in between classes. Most unnerving, a short time later I began to have trouble feeling my foot on the pedals when I drove. Pretty soon I was hobbling around like an infirm ninety-year-old woman.

At first I wasn't that concerned, because it wasn't unusual for me to experience joint pain when I would get my period. It could get so bad that I wasn't able to play the piano for a few days, something I did regularly when my metacarpals weren't on fire. I came in an hour early to school each day just to play in the music room, since moving around as a kid, I didn't have regular access to a piano. I remember my disappointment at sitting down and discovering that my hands had become a clumsy mess against the keys.

I continued to ignore my symptoms, assuming I was overtired, or stressed, or perhaps anemic from my heavy periods. It wasn't until my friends started commenting on the way I was walking that I started to worry—clearly I wasn't compensating as well as I'd thought. I started having to walk the long way through the halls to class in order to use the accessible ramp, because I couldn't get up the stairs. The first few times, my friends thought it was funny. After about a week, they began to suggest that I should see a doctor.

Clearly, I should have been a lot more unsettled by the fact that, over the course of a few months, I had gradually been losing the use of my legs. I found it curious, but not disturbing. I was certain that there was a logical explanation for it; therefore, it caused me no real anxiety. If I didn't give it the power to frighten me, then it wouldn't. That's what I told myself, anyway.

My regular doctor referred me to a neurologist, and that's why I dutifully reported to patient registration at the hospital that morning after signing myself out of school (a privilege that I could have abused as an emancipated minor, but never did). The woman behind the desk eyed me uncertainly and asked where my parent or guardian was, since I was still a minor.

"I'm legally emancipated," I mumbled, pulling the tattered copy of my emancipation papers from my bag. "And I have Mainecare," I added, sliding the card across her desk. This was the state's Medicaid program, which I'd qualified for after a few rousing trips to the Department of Health and Human Services. I was quickly learning that no one likes Medicaid. Health-care professionals hate it because they get stiffed on payments. Many of them won't accept it, because they know they'll be underpaid for their services. Beneficiaries know that they'll inevitably be denied treatment, shamed for their "reliance on government benefits," and forced to jump through hoops to get, and keep, their coverage.

The registrar looked down the bridge of her nose at me, and I wondered if she knew what emancipation even meant.

"Really," she said—in the way an adult might feign interest in a child's nonsensical story when what they really want is a stiff drink—"Well, I still need to call your parents."

"No, um. Actually—you don't," I sputtered, feeling my face warm at the prospect of being perceived as talking back. "I don't live with them. I haven't lived with them for five years. If you call the probate court they'll fax you a fresh copy of this paperwork if you don't believe me—"

She reached for the phone, "You're a minor, so, we need your parents to—"

"My birthday is in a week," I pleaded, attempting to stare her down, "I'll be eighteen. Please. Don't call my parents. It's not legally necessary, I'm not lying," I felt tears burning my eyes, my heart strangling my throat. I willed myself not to cry, but the panic had set in, and I knew that the torrent would come.

"Don't you want your parents to know you're here?" she asked, completely indifferent to the fact that I'd just told her I hadn't lived with them in five years.

"No, you don't understand—"

"You're not a foster kid, are you? Do you have foster parents?"

"No, I'm emancipated, I'm on my own. I mean, I have someone who kind of looks after me, I guess? Her name is Estelle. She lives a few blocks away. I can give you her number—"

"Is she your guardian?"

"No! I'm my own guardian!" I snapped, finally beginning to cry. I was humiliated, and I watched powerlessly as she dialed my parents' home phone number, which must have been in my record from when I had been brought in for a strep test as a child.

"We have your daughter Abigail here and we need your consent to treat her," I heard the woman say, having presumably gotten my mother on the line. It was midmorning, so my dad would have been at work.

Hot tears ran down my face and I felt my legs begin to shake. It was strangely reassuring, because I hadn't exactly been feeling them for a few days. Now I could at least feel the sensation of my knee hitting the underside of the registration desk.

"I see," the woman said, eyeing me, "Well, thank you." She hung up the phone, grabbed my emancipation papers, and stood up. "I'll be right back, I need to make a copy of these."

I pulled myself together while she was back at the copier, straightening my spine and drying my eyes on the sleeve of my sweater. My legs continued to quake, and I pressed the palms of my hands hard against my upper thighs to try to stop them.

The woman returned a few minutes later with my hospital ID bracelet and pointed me toward the lab as though nothing had happened. I thanked her, struggled to stand up, and limped out of the office down the hall.

The neurologist was completely unfazed by the specifics of my history or my alleged physical condition. I half expected myself that it was all psychological. If I'd learned anything from taking Advanced Placement Psychology the year before as a junior, it was that hysteria often manifested itself with dramatic bouts of paralysis. Maybe the stress of my weird childhood was trying to figure out which part of my body it wanted to live in. I didn't exactly give this theory to the neurologist, but I prepared myself to hear that it was all in my head.

He did a brief neurological exam, which was unremarkable except that he found it curious that I struggled to get up from a squatted position. I didn't disagree; it did feel like a struggle. He harrumphed through the rest of the exam and, doing his due diligence, I suppose, ordered more blood tests and a full-body MRI. Humoring me with a more thorough investigation in no way reassured me that he didn't think I was hysteric, but I suppose it was a step up from the historical approach of attributing such a diagnosis to a woman willy-nilly. Something I'd been enlightened about in my psych class the previous year, via the usual literature, starting with notable cases like that of Anna O.

THE CASE OF ANNA O., by Sigmund Freud and his colleague Josef Breuer, is one of the most famous psychological case studies, period—hysteria notwithstanding. While she's most often associated with Freud's body of work, she was seen by Breuer, who only conferred with Freud once he found himself unable to help her. "She was deranged," Breuer said, adding that he hoped she would die to end her suffering. The young woman they'd call Anna when they wrote up her case was twenty-one years old when she met Breuer in 1880. In *Studies on Hysteria*, on which the two psychiatrists collaborated, Anna is described as being remarkably intelligent, if not gifted, as well as kind and highly empathetic. She was, they said, capable of rational thought, and not suggestible in the least—although she did have an "astonishingly underdeveloped" sexuality. Anna, the men wrote, was "bubbling over with intellectual vitality," but leading an extremely boring life, one that was primarily devoted to caring for her ill father. Anna's own illness was presumed to be a manifestation of her anxieties, thwarted potential, and stifled sexuality. She told stories of her life—which were really stories of herself—to Breuer in the form of talk therapy, which at the time was dubbed the "talking cure."

Despite the initial grim prognosis, Anna O.—whose real name was Bertha Pappenheim—made a full recovery, having committed to this kind of emotional work. Whether she was working through past traumas or current anxieties, her physical and mental symptoms resolved once attention was paid to them. She went on to have a very successful career as a social worker, becoming the founder of the Jewish Women's Association.

It's no wonder that she became a textbook case: her diagnosis was fairly straightforward and responded to treatment. She either didn't have any underlying comorbidities, or if she did, they weren't significant enough to complicate her course. The use of psychodynamic therapy, such as the talking cure, would be complex enough, given every patient's unique emotional experiences and perspectives; add in physical pathologies (known and unknown), and it becomes a much more complex task. And that initial focus on the emotional state, or the preference for ascribing a psychiatric explanation to a physical presentation, may well lead to a misdiagnosis.

In 1962, when she was seventeen years old, two notable things happened to Karen Armstrong: she joined a convent, and she began having fainting spells. In her book *The Spiral Staircase*, she eloquently discusses her emotional and spiritual journey, but also gives vital weight to the concurrent physical maladies that plagued her. The spells that she had were not just peculiar and alarming, but embarrassing. The nuns in the convent often told her she needed to pull herself together, or accused her of being melodramatic. She even recalled entertaining the assumption herself as she attempted to come up with an explanation for the bizarre symptoms: "I assumed that even though I might not be feeling especially upset, I was displaying some subconscious need for notice, love, or intimacy. The blackouts, I concluded, must be a bid for attention."

No one so much as suggested she visit the infirmary, let alone see a doctor. She was assumed, by others, even eventually by herself, to be weak-willed—or malevolently manipulative—for years before anyone gave credence to the idea that she might be ill. She eventually left the convent. Had she—like Anna O. before her—been experiencing her "fits" as a result of feeling stifled by her environment, you'd think her spells would have ended. They did not, and in fact, they had been progressively worsening. Her doctor suggested that her anxiety, as he perceived her condition, needed to be treated through psychoanalysis, which she diligently undertook, although she had doubts: "I would be overtaken by a queasy sense of déjà vu. This was exactly the sort of reasoning that I had used in the convent, and look where it had got me."

It had been nearly a decade since she'd joined the convent and begun experiencing the fainting spells, the progressively worsening blackouts, and lost time. And she had, in fact, lost a lot of time. Years of her young life, nearly her entire twenties, were marred by the symptoms and the fruitless quest to explain them, let alone cure them. Then, one day nearly fifteen years after that quest had begun, she ended up in the emergency room after a particularly bad spell. When she woke up, she was told she'd had a grand mal seizure, and was referred to a neurologist at once.

She regaled the neurologist with the story of her years of symptoms, and he asked her why she had not gone to a doctor about them, when they were clearly so troubling and serious. Oh, but she had, she said. She explained to him that she'd been seeing doctors for years. The doctor was stunned into what she called a "devastating quiet" before asking her if any of them, when she had told them of these symptoms (which he felt were demonstrative of a "textbook case" of temporal lobe epilepsy), had ever suggested she have an electroencephalogram (EEG) of her brain.

No, she told him. They had not.

While it was enraging enough that her symptoms had automatically been assumed to have no physical origin, the fact that a fairly simple test was not done to even attempt to disprove that theory outraged Armstrong's doctor. Her condition was not particularly uncommon, and it was not even necessarily going to be difficult to treat. Had someone identified it when she was in her late teens (*precisely* when that form of epilepsy often presents for the first time because of the hormonal change associated with puberty), it never would have gained that much power over her life.

—※—

I WAS ABOUT THE SAME age as Armstrong when her journey began when I had my first MRI to more closely examine my classically hysterical symptom of leg weakness. I suppose now I'm grateful that the test was even ordered, but at the time, as the technician injected me with a dye that made my whole arm feel hot, and that gave me a heady, woozy feeling as I was sucked back into the giant, obstreperous tube, I just felt very alone. I lay there feeling incredibly hollow, although there was something oddly calming about being in such a small space (luckily I'm not the least bit claustrophobic).

I considered that perhaps when I left for Sarah Lawrence in the fall I wouldn't be able to dance. Maybe I'd have to give up the piano. But whatever happened, I was confident that it wouldn't slow me down. It couldn't. I had worked too hard for it to all go to shambles just because my legs were a little wobbly. I simply refused to acknowledge the possibility that I wouldn't be able to do what I wanted to do when I graduated from high school a few months later.

I started out with a lot of faith in medical science, despite all the ways it had failed my mother when I was growing up. If there was something wrong with me, it would be different. I would get well, because I wanted to be well, and I would simply do whatever it took. Surgery, therapy, drugs—whatever was required, I'd do it. I had no fear, because I trusted that doctors knew how to fix people—so long as they wanted to be fixed.

My mother remained ill because she wanted to be ill.

That's what I convinced myself, anyway. I followed up with the neurologist a few weeks after my birthday, which made things considerably easier. Having become of legal age, I didn't have to go through the same traumatic registration protocol as before. The doctor explained that the MRI was more or less fine—there were some incidentally discovered structural oddities that were probably congenital and nothing to worry about.

While I was relieved that there wasn't anything gravely wrong with me, I was a bit irked that the doctor had offered nothing to make my legs work right again. I had thought that, at the very least, he could give me some kind of medication that would fix the wobbly feelings and let me get my life back. He thought the situation was strange, but he had no answer. He figured he would follow up in a few months to see if it had gotten any worse. Though I simmered with impatience, I accepted this and vowed to do whatever I needed to do to make sure these annoying symptoms didn't get in my way any longer. If it meant I had to go down stairs on my butt, I would. At times, that's exactly what I did.

Over the course of the next several months, the strange symptoms gradually got better. By midsummer they had all but resolved. I still had some trouble that correlated with my menstrual cycle, but I laughed it off as my personal misfortune. It had taken about six months, all and all, but I had finally regained a normal gait. When I arrived at Sarah Lawrence in the fall, I headed to dance class undeterred.

When I got sick, after only being there a little over a year, I didn't make any kind of connection, and when I went to the hospital in Bronxville, I never even mentioned the earlier problem. It hadn't occurred to me to.

Finding myself back in Maine about eighteen months later, in that very same hospital, at the same registration booth even—the memories reached for me like keening banshees. As I walked down the hall toward the lab, I did entertain the idea that these two experiences might be connected—but almost immediately shook the thought from my mind. There had been nothing wrong then. The doctor had said so, hadn't he? And maybe it had taken half a year, but eventually I had gotten better.

And whatever was happening to me now was far worse anyway. I'd lost a great deal of weight and though the discomfort of weak, wobbly legs had been annoying, it wasn't anywhere near as bad as this constant, unrelenting pain. This time I couldn't ignore the fact that I was sick. I couldn't tell myself that nothing was wrong, because something clearly was. And I don't know what made me feel worse: the fact that I was really sick, or that I wasn't strong enough mentally to deny it.

⁓✲⁓

AFTER I LEFT SCHOOL, I saw a gynecologist, Dr. Paulson. It seemed like a logical place to go next: my periods had always been hellacious, and if the experience I'd had at school was indicative of an ovarian cyst, I thought maybe there was some kind of syndrome or predisposition that could explain it. I had been referred to Dr. Paulson by my regular Maine doctor, and she was the first gynecologist I'd seen for the problem.

I suspect that all OB/GYN offices look alike, with the same posters of smiling babies in the bathroom watching you while you struggle to collect a urine sample, the same soft pastel color schemes, the same cushy chairs for uncomfortably pregnant women. And also the same cold stirrups, plastic vagina models, and blisteringly obvious red sharps containers.

In Dr. Paulson's office I underwent two types of ultrasounds—the kind that pregnant women get, when they dollop some goo on the lower abdomen, and the internal kind. Transvaginal ultrasounds are brilliant technology, but they hurt like a bitch. I had already experienced several painful internal exams, and no matter how gentle Dr. Paulson's technician was trying to be, it was immediately clear that this experience wasn't going to be much better. On my second visit, she offered to let me guide the wand into my own vagina, which didn't hurt any less and made me furiously blush, as if I were in some kind of low-budget porn film.

These ultrasounds revealed nothing. Still, my symptoms worsened. A few months earlier, when I'd first returned to Maine and had been seen by my regular doctor, I'd mentioned that I had altogether stopped having a period. I'd also recalled, going back through my memory of the months that had led up to the incident in the shower, that prior to that I'd experienced several weeks of bleeding that appeared to have no cause. Strangely, it was all what you might call "old" blood, though: brown clots that ruined my underwear, not to mention one very nice leotard of which I'd been particularly fond. I suspected that maybe this was all somehow connected, but only in retrospect. At the time, I'd been more annoyed than anything else. I certainly hadn't expected it to culminate in something quite so disabling.

My doctor had listened to this, and when she'd written the referral to Dr. Paulson, it was for a surgical consult for "probable endometriosis," often referred to as "endo." She'd written that assessment in the margin of her office notes—but hadn't so much as said it aloud to me in the office, let alone explained it. I was put on a drug called Provera that would chemically force me to have a period. Force me it did.

Medroxyprogesterone is a synthetic form of the hormone progesterone, which helps regulate ovulation and, therefore, the menstrual cycle. Depo-Provera, another form of the drug but in much higher doses, is given as an injection for birth control. I was prescribed a relatively small dose, one 5 milligram pill each day for ten days, and when my period finally started it felt like several months' worth of periods all at once. I bled heavily and for a long time. When I went in for my diagnostic laparoscopy with Dr. Paulson, I still hadn't stopped bleeding.

On the morning of my surgery, Cass, a beloved high school teacher with whom I had formed a very close bond, came to my aid, along with my best friend, Hillary. I had never had surgery before, and I was worried about where I would go to recover. The three of us sat crunched into a curtained partition in pre-op, and I brushed off my nonstop shaking as I got undressed. The hospital had an airy chill, but the truth was that I was scared.

Hillary and I were joking around in the surgical suite when the nurse came in and announced that she needed to shave me for surgery. I didn't know what she meant. Did they really care if my legs weren't shaved? When she suggested Hillary and Cass might want to go on the other side of the privacy curtain, I realized she meant she was going to shave my pubic region, which came as a complete shock to me. That hadn't been in the pre-op survey.

In retrospect, I kind of wish they'd given me the sedative first, because it was pretty humiliating. I hadn't had a serious boyfriend yet, so no one had ever seen my pubes before—other than my gynecologist, and she hadn't thrown in a bikini wax along with my last pap smear. Thank God Hillary was on the other side of that curtain— laughing in her contagious, boisterous way—otherwise I would have been crying from embarrassment rather than from laughing every time she popped her head around the corner of the curtain to check the progress of my pubic topiary.

The anesthesiologist came in to sedate me, and Cass and Hillary were sequestered away to the waiting room. There was a moment between Hillary and me when the laughter subsided, and we looked at one another with fear: What if I wasn't okay? She tried to hide her tears, but I knew she was scared too.

I remember being taken to the operating room. It looked pretty much exactly like the ORs on TV, but it was frigidly cold—this time, my teeth were chattering because I was actually cold rather than frightened. I climbed off the gurney and onto the operating table, which felt really weird, and definitely not how they would have done it on *Grey's Anatomy*. I remember the mask being put over my face, the nurse telling me to count backwards from ten—and my first thought was, *Oh, I have to make it to one! How crazy would that be? Would I win something? I don't even feel that slee—*

I woke up several hours later. The surgery had taken twice as long as Dr. Paulson had anticipated because of what she'd discovered. Cass and Hillary had been beside themselves while I'd been blissfully unaware on the table, then dozing in recovery. Because I'd been pumped full of intravenous Zofran and painkillers following the surgery, I later remembered only a few things that Dr. Paulson said. Luckily, Cass and Hillary were able to fill in the gaps. The few words that I caught—torqued tube, chocolate cyst, spots of endometriosis— seemed like some kind of an answer, at least. I remember her apologizing, saying that she "didn't know how they'd missed it on an ultrasound"—"it" being the large cyst that had displaced my ovary. It was, in fact, larger than—and blooped out from—the fimbria of my left fallopian tube.

The fimbriae are the little fingers that waggle and grab onto the egg when it pops out of the ovary. They then guide the egg into the opening of the fallopian tube, where it be-bops down into the uterus. This cyst I had on the end of this tube's fimbria was so large that it had twisted the tube itself, sort of backward, behind my uterus. In the photos it looks sort of like when you wring out a washcloth.

Dr. Paulson explained to me that these ovoid-like structures are often referred to as "chocolate cysts" because they're filled with old, brown blood that looks like, well, chocolate syrup. So, first of all—*yuck*.

I assumed this all meant that she had removed the ovary and possibly even the tube, but she had not. Instead, she had just drained the cyst and wrapped it, and my fallopian tube, with something called Interceed, a kind of surgical fabric that is eventually supposed to be absorbed into the body. Surgical mess can sometimes cause adhesions (as can endometriosis, incidentally). She wouldn't have been able to remove the cyst without disrupting the ovary, and likely the tube as well. I took that as gospel. It never occurred to me to ask if someone else might have been able—or willing—to remove it all. Such a choice would have impacted my fertility—which somehow took precedence over everything else in her eyes, including my pain, despite the fact that I would never have had even the remotest qualm about subfertility, a fact that I have always tried to make clear to any medical professional ever since. I can only assume that doctors don't feel comfortable taking a woman's word for it when she says she's not concerned about her fertility, and that they insist on preserving it to avoid later lawsuits. I was slowly figuring out that not only was my pain going to be disbelieved, but it was never going to take precedence.

Dr. Paulson had also mentioned that she had found "endometriosis" on the wall behind my uterus. It was another word, like "Interceed," that didn't really mean much to me at first. I assumed it was probably something congenital—some weird thing I'd been born with because I had been a Very Hungry Fetus and therefore hadn't developed properly. She didn't explain, and I didn't ask, because I was still sedated—but she left me with her confidence that, having drained the cyst, she felt that I would begin to feel better. She'd see me in her office for follow-up in a few weeks.

I was discharged shortly thereafter, and for the first few days all I did was sleep. When I woke up, my stitches were sore, but that was a pain I had expected. I held out hope that once the incision healed, I wouldn't have pain at all. That whatever had happened to me, it was behind me now, and that I'd soon get the all-clear to go back to Sarah Lawrence and resume my life—which had only paused, not stopped.

My follow-up appointment with Dr. Paulson was brief: I asked her if I'd be well enough to go back to school now that she'd taken care of this problematic cyst. She'd said *probably*. I balked—what did she mean, *probably*? Wasn't I better?

She calmly explained that the cyst might come back. Or, it might not. If it did come back, it might be in a couple of months, a year, a few years. It took me a minute to process what she was saying, but when it hit me, I felt like I'd been gutted: this could happen again.

I had naïvely assumed that I was fixed. It seemed logical enough: I'd gotten sick, I'd gone to the doctor, and it had taken a few rather long, dark months, but it seemed that an answer had been found. I'd had surgery, and now—what? I was being told that it might just happen all over again? In retrospect, that was the moment I realized that my ignorance was going to exacerbate whatever the problem was, and that I had to prescribe myself some kind of medical education, at least as it pertained to my situation.

Dr. Paulson said that after the next few weeks, as the last of my stitches dissolved, I'd have a pretty clear idea of whether I felt better enough to go back to school. If I did, she'd certainly clear me for that. It was a gamble, but ultimately, the decision was up to me.

I was still holding out hope. I tried to lightly exercise my body as much as my healing scars permitted. I missed dancing and stretching and moving. I dreamt of being back at school most nights, and often woke up in the morning somewhat disoriented by not being there anymore.

⸺❀⸺

GIVEN THE INTENSITY OF MY introspective analysis during those long winter months, it's no surprise that I remember the exact moment

I realized the fight wasn't over—that it had never really ended. I was sitting on the couch at Cass's house after everyone had gone back to school or work after Christmas (and I had not gone back anywhere other than the depths of my own despair), watching reruns of *The X-Files*, which had been my favorite show since childhood.

The X-Files is not, by any stretch, a children's show. But when I was about eight or nine and mostly free from parental supervision, I'd stumbled across it one night when I couldn't sleep. It was dark and atmospheric, with this inexplicable beauty in its carefully constructed tension. I found it soothing: the perpetual feeling of nighttime, whispers, a sense of intimacy that made it feel more like reading a book than watching TV. It could be a truly gory, frightening show—and no child should have been lulled to sleep by those images. But even with its heaviness, I liked knowing that even if I fell asleep before the episode was over, the heroes, Agents Mulder and Scully, would keep going. That they would still be out there somewhere, searching for the truth. Even if no one believed in it or in them.

At first I liked Mulder the best, because he reminded me of my father. My dad had the same coloring and bone structure as David Duchovny, and my child's mind imagined my father as some kind of alternate-universe, blue-collar, rugged, steel-toed-boot Mulder.

By the time I was a teen, I'd become a bona fide X-Phile—Internet fan forums and all. Given my proclivity for suits, science, and "sticking it to the Man," I had come to idolize the character of Dana Scully. She demonstrated a complexity that, as I've grown up, I've found the world does not easily accept—in women, at least. Even now, I find myself looking to Scully for a reminder that it's okay for women to be contrarians. That women can be smart, and tough, competent, and still be afraid, or feel their feelings all-consumingly, or demonstrate femininity in whatever capacity they desire. That these things are not inherently mutually exclusive, and that they are not defined for you by the men in your life. You can take down a global government conspiracy in heels and use your perfectly manicured fingernails to gouge out the eyes of a would-be murderer.

Upon re-watching the series throughout my recovery, I realized that what I had internalized of Scully—her skepticism, her doggedness, her curiosity and intelligence—were largely the parts of myself that I was proud of and loved. They were also, consequently, very much under siege. Those attributes had, at times, been compromised for Scully, too—by illness or injury or shadowy government conspiracies. She always grieved her losses (of which both she and Mulder experienced many) and carried on. She fought her way through the pain. I thought about that a lot as I sat on Cass's couch, figuratively licking my emotional wounds as my literal surgical wounds wept into their dressings.

Then, as I was watching, a familiar feeling crept into my pelvis. A peculiar pang under my hip bone. A deep, nauseating ache that was not the superficial pain of surgical scars. Nor was it akin to the gas pains that lingered in the first week or so after my procedure.

No, this pain was insidious. This pain was new—except it wasn't. This pain had struck me down the season before and consumed me. This was a pain that I knew. A pain that I had hoped to forget. I sat motionless, completely alone in that big farmhouse, crying quietly as I closed my eyes and tried to convince myself it wasn't happening. Just talk yourself out of it, I pleaded with myself, trying to reason that it couldn't be the same pain. It had to be something else.

I went full skeptical Scully on my body, coming up with every reason that it wasn't that pain. It was just a passing feeling, surely. It wouldn't last. There was no enduring mystery, no shadow stalking me, no conspiracy. My body was not frantically destroying itself in service to corporeal paranoia, in the form of some kind of weaponized autoimmunity.

My body was not an X-File. I would still get to go back to Sarah Lawrence. I would get better. This pain would end.

Not unlike my fictional heroes, I was about to become embroiled in a search for a truth that many did not believe was out there to be found. Like Mulder, I wanted to believe. But unlike Mulder, and more like Scully, what I wanted to believe in was science. I'd had one of Scully's quotes pinned to the inside of my locker in high school. It had gone with me to New York and back again, and it came to me that afternoon on Cass's couch: "Nothing happens in contradiction to nature, only in contradiction to what we know of it. And that's a place to start. That's where the hope is."

⸺⧉⸺

THE PREEMINENT RESEARCH ON ENDOMETRIOSIS started in the 1980s, led by an esteemed surgeon named Dr. David Redwine. Shortly before his retirement in 2012, he gave a presentation on the subject at the Endometriosis Foundation of America's annual medical conference (which I would later speak at myself). I didn't know much about him or his work, but I liked that he talked about astronomy in his speech: his title was "Asteroid Mapping, HOX Genes and Endometriosis."

Redwine likened the mapping of constellations in the night sky to his development of a way to map the pelvis in order to identify locations where endometriosis may be likely to occur. He developed the pelvic mapping based on the thousands of surgeries he performed on women with "endo," and he continued to question the veracity of the prevailing theory by gynecologist John Sampson, which was developed in the 1920s. "Sampson's theory," as it is called, purported that menstrual effluent could essentially "backwash" from the uterus, through the fallopian tubes, and out into the pelvis, where it would then implant itself as endometriosis. The rupture of a blood-filled endometrioma—or cyst, like the one I had—would have a similar capacity, according to his theory. Although the theory was presented nearly a century ago, it's never been irrefutably proven, despite the advances of medical technology that would arguably make it possible to do so, if there were substantial interest and investment.

Despite the passage of time and the ensuing progression of medical science, neither are medical textbooks overflowing with high-definition imagery of endometriosis. Although Redwine and others have pointed out that research regarding endometriosis has been happening for at least the past century, every medical textbook I've ever thumbed through (hundreds, at various hospitals, libraries, and medical centers around the United States) seems to demarcate the condition as being relatively uninteresting: even in textbooks entirely devoted to reproductive endocrinology or gynecologic surgery, the passages on endometriosis are short. They usually contain the same refrain about how endometriosis is a disease of the female reproductive system where cells from inside the uterus wind up in places that they shouldn't. Infertility is usually the bolded point of interest. The litany of facts presented, even in the more contemporary texts I've read, sometimes seem bloated to me. These passages can read like college term papers written the night before they're due, wherein a lot of unnecessary words are added to make the paper longer.

You'd think that after reading thousands of pages about endometriosis I'd feel like I know a lot. But I don't. I feel like I know the same facts and theories very well, but I have been left with an abundance of questions. Some of which are questions that science and medicine appear to be interested in, even if just for the sake of academic conference discourse: Have women always been vulnerable to endometriosis? Were cavewomen staggering around in pain? Can disciplines like anthropology and archeology give us insight? Were those Victorian hysterics suffering from adhesions and cysts? If history had been told by women, would we not be so in the dark about a disease that has, theoretically, always existed? Is the mechanism of disease a product of menstruation? Or is something else key to its development? Does it matter where you're born and raised, or where your family moved when you were a teen? Is it even possible to unspool all the factors, like genetics, environment, and diet, that influence our state of health in general, let alone the influence it may have on one specific condition? Is endometriosis preventable? Inevitable?

To whom can we look for answers? Whom can we trust? Our doctors? Doctors writing on the Internet? Doctors speaking at conferences, like Redwine? Or perhaps we can trust the researchers cited in those talks, and the alphabet soup of sources appearing in medical journals. How do I, as a patient, know what to believe, what to build my life upon with this disease? As a young woman writing this book, which can never be comprehensive and is merely trying to put my own experience into context, how am I to know if the information I've relied upon in my quest for answers is the "right" information?

We don't know much about endometriosis. If you compare what we know about other diseases that affect around the same number of people as endometriosis (such as liver disease), you find that the amount of information we don't know is startling. If you put "endometriosis" into PubMed, you get about 1,800 pages of results. Liver disease returns over 30,000.

The scientific and medical establishment doesn't know much about endometriosis—really, it's the patients who tend to have their pulses on the most current research. Although sometimes that back-fires. A patient's main motivation for becoming an expert in his or her condition is to manage it—perhaps even cure it. The patient isn't trying to subvert his or her physician. But a frantic patient who has brought in a heap of research is often chastised, and usually advised to refrain from consulting Google. In the case of endometriosis, it's shortsighted to cast aside the engaged and eager patient: What physician has the time to review all the current literature on a particular condition? A patient who is trying take an active role in her care will use whatever tools she has available to her within the limitations of her life, limitations that are often determined largely by her disease, her socioeconomic circumstances, and her level of education.

The patient who brings in a binder full of PubMed articles should be considered not so much for the specifics of what she has found, but for the fact that she has devoted so much time to the search. It may not be that the research she has brought is pertinent, or, at that particular time, even useful. But the very act of researching, and of supplying the fruits of that quest, is clinically relevant, if only because they are evidence of how the condition has affected the patient's life. I say this as a patient who researched as though my life depended on it. Which I suppose it did. Had the physicians who tutted at my eagerness, at my intellectual intensity, at my DIY medical school education, read between the lines, they would have seen the stacks of medical textbooks next to my bed, and the hundreds of bookmarked articles with up-to-date information, as a symptom of the anxiety that endometriosis caused me. I wasn't just seeking answers to absolve the pain; I was trying to soothe the fears that stemmed from the uncertainty of it.

I'm certain that not every endometriosis patient, or every chronically ill patient, for that matter, presents this way. I'm certain that not every patient cares about the whys or hows or what fors. Not every patient will be thrown into an existential crisis trying to find answers to the mysteries of their own bodies. Those who do, like me, are trying to process their physical experience in an intellectual manner. For me, it was in part because I was afraid of fully embodying what it meant to feel unwell. To feel pain. I focused on unraveling the scientific basis of my situation so that I could feel detached from it. I was also seeking answers and trying to give meaning to my suffering.

I was also, I think, trying to assuage my guilt. As much as I was looking for a reason, or a treatment, or a cure, I was also looking for proof that the disease was purely physical, and not some kind of cosmic punishment. I needed concrete evidence of rogue cells, of inflammation, of scars and blood and twisted fascia. I needed to understand, fully, the science of inflammation. I clung to the concepts of cytokines, telocytes, interleukins, and genetic polymorphisms because, if I could make them complicit, I could exonerate myself. Blame had been circling me since I had gotten sick, waiting for me to pause long enough for it to devour me. I'd come to feel, deep down in that tangled mess of organs, that the disease was my fault. And no matter how much I searched for evidence to the contrary, it didn't seem like medicine could entirely prove me wrong. In fact, a lot of people in my life—doctors, psychologists, others—left me feeling responsible. I was frigid, tense, too stressed, too smart for my own good, didn't have enough fun. Was I searching for an identity in disease? Trying to avoid sex? Fearful of intimacy? Desperate for attention?

I had no way to defend myself, really. I didn't think endometriosis was truly a mysterious disease for which there were no answers; science just wasn't there yet. And until science got there, I would have to endure the doubt. Doubt being a comorbidity with a symptom profile and treatment protocol, a prognosis all its own.

We don't know, with any degree of certainty, how or why endometriosis begins. We don't know why some women get it and others do not. We don't know why some women get it, suffer, and then appear to stop suffering at certain points in their lives. We don't know why a woman with only a few scattered lesions might have debilitating symptoms and a woman who is chock-full of them might feel fine.

Even the textbook facts are not widely agreed upon. The doctor you see, his or her level of experience, and to some extent gender, will determine how endometriosis is explained to you. Some will tell you there's no cure. Some will say there is a cure, but they can't provide it. There are plenty of surgeons who could be staring right at endometrial lesions and would not recognize them. There are a few surgeons who are experienced in excising the lesions, and some women have felt that after that procedure, they've been cured. Some women who had the touted curative surgery did not feel cured—either because the disease came back, or because some of the lesions were missed the first time around. (According to Dr. Redwine, the research indicates that the cure rate for excision surgeries is around 56 to 66 percent.)

Not every patient has access to excision surgery. I, for one, was never offered it, and it was only through discussions with other patients that I learned about it. I also learned that the surgeons who did it had very long wait lists and didn't take my insurance. If excision surgery is, as a matter of scientific fact, curative, what does it matter to me if I can't access it? And what if that fact doesn't help me? Do I need permission to push beyond the realm of present scientific fact and look for other possibilities that are within my reach? Is it appropriate, or valuable, for me to assert that possibilities might well exist within my body, or my mind, and that those stagnant facts in perennially outdated textbooks aren't helpful to me? That they may not be very helpful to a lot of people with this disease? Many of whom are never given "the facts" in the first place?

Doctors who are not surgeons—or endometriosis-familiar surgeons—often discuss endometriosis as though it were incidental. They might offer birth control, a course or two of Lupron, or simply advise a patient to get pregnant: both because they believe, incorrectly, that pregnancy is curative, and because they think endometriosis is a fast-track to infertility. Some will say that a complete hysterectomy is the only option—not unlike those nineteenth-century physicians who saw castration as the cure-all for their hysteric patients. I suspect that many doctors confronted with a patient who ultimately has endometriosis says, and does, nothing at all—simply because a diagnosis of endometriosis just isn't on their radar. When you consider that many physicians practicing today, who received the bulk of their medical education prior to the 1980s, only saw endometriosis as a footnote in a textbook, I don't think we should be that surprised.

A lot of commonly held beliefs about endometriosis, by the medical profession and the general public, are based in half-truths, or in ideas that were once regarded as true, but were later proved to be false, or at least mostly false, or probably false. Such as the idea that endometriosis lesions come from inside the uterus, and that they are made of the same sort of tissue that lines the womb. And the idea that this tissue is expelled out of the fallopian tubes and into the pelvic cavity, where it implants and causes a ruckus.

The idea that they are the same sort of tissue is sort of true, according to one popular theory. The problem is that these lesions are not identical to what is found inside the uterus. As Dr. Redwine pointed out in his lecture, endometriosis lesions are not "autografts," which just means that they aren't identical to the tissue from which they came. Under a microscope, endometriosis lesions can be inspected and seen to be stromal cells, and yes, stromal cells are also found in the lining of the uterus. But these same sorts of lesions have been found in other places—such as the liver, lungs, and diaphragm—which implies that there is another mechanism of movement that determines how they get there.

I, for one, have often wondered whether the curious neck and shoulder pain I get during the first few days of my period could be related to endo somehow. I'd assumed that any musculoskeletal pain during my cycle was hormone related, which is a fairly well-documented phenomenon even in people who don't have endometriosis. But many a Google search turned up discussion forums where others described the same cyclic neck and shoulder pain, only to find out it was related to endometriosis of the diaphragm.

Now, unless your fallopian tubes are shooting out uterine tissue like a pressure washer, how else could you possibly develop lesions in such remote locations? How do you explain women who have endometrial lesions on their brain, or the backs of their eyeballs?

The theory that uterine tissue can sort of seep out of your fallopian tubes and end up in places it doesn't belong is called *retrograde menstruation*. And, in fact, pretty much anyone who has ever menstruated has probably had some of this menstrual backwash before. What usually happens is that your body recognizes that the tissue doesn't belong, and wipes it up. Your immune system should respond to that uterine tissue in your pelvic cavity like, "What is this mess? Really? I let you live here rent-free and you can't even pick up after yourself? How hard is it to keep the mess contained to your own damn space. Honest to God, . . ." so muttering as it reluctantly mops up the mess.

The human immune system is like the TV sitcom mom of yore who begrudgingly cleans up the messes of the rest of the family. So when an autoimmune disease occurs, it's kind of like your internal immune-mother goes full Thelma and Louise and bails on you without so much as a casserole in the freezer.

Researchers are curious about what, if any, interplay exists between endometriosis and the autoimmune system. Is endometriosis something that occurs because of a compromised autoimmune system, or does the presence of endometriosis lead to autoimmune dysfunction?

The link between endometriosis and fertility, meanwhile, is less about causation and more about correlation. Endometriosis is more likely to be diagnosed in women who are infertile because those women are seeking treatment since they can't get pregnant. This doesn't mean that women with endometriosis are doomed to infertility, and in fact, recent cohort studies see a much smaller correlation than is typically espoused. Endometriosis—particularly advanced stage disease in women who have never undergone any kind of surgical treatment—could certainly contribute to infertility structurally. But many women with endometriosis are able to get pregnant and go on to have normal, uncomplicated births.

The current model of staging endometriosis is often criticized because it has an arbitrary point system for classification, which is fantastically short-sighted when you consider that the disease can cause such debilitating symptoms. Staging other chronic diseases, such as multiple sclerosis, factors in not only test results but also quality-of-life indicators or episodes of symptoms. Flare-ups of multiple sclerosis can take on different timetables, too—being "relapsing-remitting," in some cases. Could endometriosis, a hormone-dependent disease, at least at the outset, also be capable of appearing on a relapsing-remitting course?

Symptoms of endometriosis can persist throughout the month, but the majority of women I've interviewed agree that the flow of symptoms is at least influenced, if not driven, by their menstrual cycle. Because of the tissue's similarities to uterine tissue, research has posited it's estrogen-dependent. Treatments that aim to suppress estrogen sometimes provide relief, but for some, when that treatment is discontinued the symptoms return. Similarly, many women find relief from their pain during pregnancy, but once the baby is born, the normal pattern of symptoms resumes.

Who are we talking about here? Who gets endometriosis? Do we even know? Some studies cite an incidence of as little as 2 percent of the general population, others of as much as 10 percent. Although the most commonly touted figure is "one in ten women," one should always refer back to the population being studied to produce that statistic. Many of these studies obtained their data by reviewing medical records for things like surgeries and hospital stays—which means the women included in their cohort are only those who had access to health care. Access to health care varies not just state to state, but even within states, and even within communities.

When studies conclude that endometriosis is a disease predominantly seen in white women, we need to be very critical of that assessment: just because the women whose hospital records were reviewed were predominantly white, that doesn't necessarily prove that more white women have endometriosis. What it tells us is that more white women are accessing health-care services. Poor women, minority women, LGBTQ persons, and people with mental or physical disabilities face significant challenges accessing health care even at the most basic level, such as for an annual physical, let alone specialists for problems like endometriosis or infertility.

Of course, we know that just because a woman has that access, it doesn't mean her concerns or symptoms will be taken seriously. But before we can even address the mistreatment that occurs once a woman is interacting with the health-care system, we have to address the fact that some women never get that far. We won't get a true picture of the incidence of endometriosis until we specifically look for it in marginalized communities. And before we can do that, we have to address the disparity in access. Social epidemiologist Jhumka Gupta has said that endometriosis is a social justice issue. In her speech at the Worldwide Endo March in Washington, DC, on March 19, 2016, she said that endometriosis is a social pathology, which she defined as "gender inequality, social injustice, and attitudes of society that keep women and girls from fully reaching their potential."

In other words, we really don't know how many people have endometriosis, and why we don't has far less to do with a lack of scientific research and advancement than with our antiquated belief systems and power structures. But it's not even that we don't understand endometriosis on a population level: we can't even seem to get it right with just one patient.

Endometriosis is so easily misdiagnosed because when symptoms do present, they can be vague, difficult to articulate, and embarrassing. It's not yet socially acceptable to announce, "I get crampy, fiery-hot diarrhea on my period!" Nor is it easy to say, "Not only is penetrative sex impossible for me, I can't even masturbate in peace because the subtle contractions of my uterus during an orgasm make my pelvis ache and not in a good way!"

The struggle to explain what endometriosis actually feels like is very real. The pain itself is of its own breed, yet it feels just similar enough to other pains that when described as such, the possible diagnoses abound. It also exists on a spectrum of severity that means that sometimes the pain level is all-consuming, and other times it's like trying to look at something in your periphery without turning your head. It's there, you know it's there, but it's like trying to catch the air around a bird's wings.

It only took a few years for the pain to just become a part of me. Suddenly, what was notable wasn't when it flared up—but when it didn't. Even now, it's been so many years since I've lived in a pain-free body that I don't really remember what it feels like.

This idea of how we experience our internal selves—physically, that is—has fascinated medicine for centuries. There's a constant hustle and bustle inside of us at any given moment: our heart beating, stomach digesting, intestines wriggling about as they do. Sometimes we're privy to this work with a twinge or a gurgle, but it's not like we feel all our internal organs. Those nineteenth-century doctors, who knew little about the workings of the nervous system, didn't find it reasonable that a woman could proclaim that she felt her uterus. And the harder she tried to explain it, the more unhinged they thought she was.

Oftentimes, that awareness of the internal workings of one's body comes about as a warning; something's not quite right. There's inflammation or injury. Usually, for the minor stuff, we can reason through it: the scratchy sore throat before a cold, the burning muscle pain after a workout, midafternoon tension headaches. These are sensations most of us are familiar with, and we can pay attention to them, articulate them to others, and conjure up those feelings in our own bodily memory when they're articulated to us.

With endo, it seems to me that those internal sensations are so poorly understood outside a woman's body (i.e., medical science) that it's extremely difficult to process it internally. The best we can do is relate it back to an experience we've had, or that we know is commonly understood: "It's sort of like period cramps, but much worse . . ."

Some women have straight-up compared it to contractions during childbirth, though they insist that endometriosis pain is worse—at least in part because it's a constant, sometimes daily endurance. Childbirth, at its most profound, is a few days of intense physical discomfort. And with childbirth, at least there's some kind of payoff: after hours upon hours of contractions, you get a baby. I can only imagine that women have long suffered childbirth with that payoff in mind.

Endometriosis has no such incentive, and for me, it began to feel like unrelenting punishment. In a metaphorical, feminist sense, I felt like there was something terribly sad about the female reproductive system attacking itself in such a way. I've always happily identified with my femininity, whether or not I was strictly a "girly-girl" by society's standards. As I struggled to understand endometriosis—and accept the limitations in that understanding—I felt strangely detached from that delight that womanhood had always brought me. In the early days, when the word "infertility" was thrown around a lot, I struggled with my lifelong devotion to childlessness. The thought of being unable to get pregnant bothered me—not because I'd wanted a child, though, but because I'd wanted a choice.

Those types of esoteric questions quickly became too much for me to think about. They were emotionally wrought, and I was exhausted in a way I couldn't seem to explain properly to anyone. It's an oppressive feeling: it's like gravity is boring down on you. This is still true for me. That kind of awareness of physical fatigue causes a parallel mental fatigue that is not limited to negative thoughts or worries—every thought seems to take a disproportionate amount of effort. Sometimes it feels like my thoughts are behind a wall of foggy glass that I have to shatter, but I don't have the strength, so I just try to wipe away the fog and squint. Once in a while I manage to crack the glass, but somehow that only obscures it more.

The pain can be like that, too. Something that I know is there, just beyond, yet that I cannot touch or soothe. Sometimes I think that if I could only look at it, I would be able to make it go away. Other times, I wonder what I would do if I found myself face-to-face with it. Would I recognize it? Would it see me?

When I was a teenager and had probably only had something like twenty periods, I was often stopped cold in my tracks by cramps. For a minute or two, I'd be frozen in time, gripped by pain, and I was forced to stare it down for those long, agonizing moments. I used to try to imagine what my uterus looked like, what the organs around it were like. I would distract myself by trying to look inside my own body. I wondered if someday, when I died, I'd be able to be a ghost in the autopsy room. If I'd see my own uterus being lifted out of my body and recognize it from my literal navel-gazing.

Back then, I didn't have a word, let alone a concept, for that pain. I didn't hear the word "endometriosis" until I was no longer a teenager. But teenagers certainly do have endometriosis, and thanks to the work of places like the Endometriosis Foundation, those young people will have a word for their pain a lot sooner than I did. In some schools, endometriosis pops up in sex ed classes now.

Although it seems that most people with endometriosis begin having symptoms at or around the time of their first period (whether they know it or not), calling endometriosis a "period problem" doesn't account for the phenomenon of endometrial lesions found in the pelvic cavities of fetuses. Fetuses who have, clearly, not menstruated. Endometriosis has been discovered during fetal autopsies, a finding that seriously challenges the widely held belief that endometriosis is strictly a menstruation-dependent disease.

Up until 2014, none of the fetal case studies reported were from the United States. That's not to say that it hadn't happened here. It's more likely that the reason it was being found elsewhere was that researchers were actively looking for it, unlike in the United States, where a more reactionary, passive approach has been taken. In the United States, this sort of approach isn't limited to reproductive medicine, but is more a reflection of the health-care system's modus operandi in general.

A case report from the American Society of Reproductive Medicine in 2015 told the story of an eighteen-year-old woman, thirty-five weeks pregnant, in whom a fetal abdominal mass was detected by ultrasound. By thirty-seven weeks, the mass had enlarged. When the baby was delivered, a surgical exploration of its pelvic and abdominal cavities revealed a large, cyst-like structure, which was removed and sent to pathology. What was it? A hemorrhagic endometrioma, with focal endometriosis. The fetus had endometriosis.

It's like *Inception*: the uterus inside the fetus (which is inside the uterus of the mother) has endometriosis. Just let that sink in for a minute.

Do the mothers of these fetuses have endometriosis? For most contemporary doctors, the fact that the patient is pregnant would probably be enough to rule out endometriosis, even though we know that endometriosis does not necessarily equal infertility.

The fact that fetuses can have endometriosis could give us remarkable insight into how the disease develops. Could it be that something happens in utero, when the uterus itself is forming, that allows that tissue to live in places it doesn't belong, even though it only typically becomes a problem once a young woman approaches puberty and begins to secrete the estrogen that the tissue needs to thrive? Dr. Redwine, clearly a system's thinker, if his constellatory map of the female pelvis is any indication, believes that endometriosis comes down to trouble with the genes responsible for executing the plan of our bodies as we develop in utero. *Homeobox* genes (also called Hox genes, because, I guess, Homeobox needed a nickname) are the genes that determine how we're built—why we have legs where we have legs and ears where we have ears. Though these genes aren't responsible for actually building limbs and organs, they do the directing—and if Hox genes possess mutations, development doesn't go according to plan. Hox genes are full of Hox proteins that are DNA enhancers, meaning they attach themselves to certain genes and either activate or repress them. Hox genes are also remarkably consistent from species to species. I have the same Hox genes as my dog and the fly on my window. The difference lies in our respective body plans: my dog's Hox genes sent her the same instructions for Hox proteins as mine did, but her body plan yielded a cute mutt and mine a circumspect brunette—with endometriosis. As Dr. Redwine explained in his lecture, he believes that Hox genes play an important role in the development of endometriosis, a process that precedes menstruation—that precedes birth, even. Abnormal differentiation of Hox genes within the developing reproductive tract gives rise to that endometrial-themed tissue manifesting in places it doesn't belong, still programmed to do its work, just in the wrong location. Sometimes, the very, very wrong location.

Dr. Redwine isn't the only person who has come to believe that endometriosis begins embryonically, but he was certainly one of the first. His original work was published in the late 1980s, and it's only been within the past decade or so that others have converged with the theory he's presented. But because it so directly challenges Sampson's theory of retrograde menstruation, which has been the primary explanation for nearly a century, whether it will sit well with clinicians (who are not always researchers) is another matter entirely. For doctors who have been using Sampson's theory (which is straightforward, easy to explain, and fairly simple for patients to comprehend) as an explanation for patients, having to grasp a more complex theory, and in turn distill it down for patient consumption, may seem a particularly daunting task. I don't know how long it typically takes for these high-level theories that exist in the realm of scientific research to trickle down into clinical practice and eventually the public consciousness—but a lack of research funding and scientific consensus certainly hasn't served to expedite what I can only assume is, at best, a somewhat lethargic process. Regretfully, such long, drawn-out processes cost people their lives; medical science can't advance quickly enough to save everyone. The casualties of the as-yet-unknowns, as with Gilda Radner, become rallying cries and warnings—even as their lives were filled with warnings that went unheeded. In *It's Always Something*, Radner wrote that she wasn't even that surprised when she found out she had ovarian cancer, because she'd always had problems with ovarian cysts. By the time medicine caught up to her, I'd wager that Radner was the one who was the least surprised by the diagnosis. What resonated with me about her story, and about Karen Armstrong's story, was the deep knowing of her own body as a woman that is seemingly unworthy of anyone's consideration or respect. I find that deeply unnerving: that I might be dying, and no one would believe me, but that feeling of inescapable truth wouldn't leave me no matter how much other people denied it.

As I FINISHED RADNER'S BOOK, I found that of all the things I would have wanted to ask her, I would have wanted to see how she felt about that denial of truth. I would have wanted to confer with her on this. Whenever people pose that question about famous dinner guests, living or dead, you'd like to entertain, Gilda's always topped my list. It'd be a Saturday night, of course. We'd sit in the middle of my living-room floor, because I tend to eschew comfort and social convention, and I feel like she did too. She'd bum a cigarette off me, then change her mind halfway through and hand it back, as we talked about dogs and tap dancing and bulimia.

I always imagine that after hours of me not being brave enough to ask her about dying, she'd take my hand and yank me up from the floor. She'd say something like, "I know you want to ask me about dying, but I want to ask you about living." She'd ask me if I'd ever laughed during sex (yes), or in church (yes), or in therapy (yes). She'd make me tell her about the time I laughed so hard I pissed my pants all over my middle-school boyfriend.

Then she'd tell me dying was like laughing so hard you don't make any sound.

CHAPTER 3

*What we needed was someone who bled . . . mothers big
enough, wide enough for us to hide in, . . . mothers who
would breathe for us when we could not breathe anymore,
who would fight for us, who would kill for us, die for us.*

—Janet Fitch, *White Oleander*

SYBIL—THE WOMAN WITH SIXTEEN personalities who was immortalized by Sally Field in the eponymous 1976 miniseries—was perhaps the most famous hysteric of the twentieth century. Sybil Dorsett lived decades after Anna O., and her story brought such horror into the public consciousness that not even Freud could have imagined it.

Sybil was not her real name. It was a name given to her by the psychiatrist, Dr. Connie Wilbur, who treated her from 1954 at least up until the book *Sybil* was published in 1973, for which the doctor enlisted the help of a writer named Flora Rheta Schreiber. Joanne Woodward portrayed Dr. Wilbur in the miniseries opposite Sally Field as Sybil, and probably many people imagine the two actresses when they hear the names. But the real Dr. Wilbur was a lot tougher than how Woodward played her. By the time Dr. Wilbur first met Shirley Ardell Mason—the girl who would become known as Sybil Isabel Dorsett—she had been fighting for years to be taken seriously as a psychologist by her male colleagues. During World War II, women had a unique opportunity to enter the workforce because so many men had been drafted. When the men returned from the war, women who had enjoyed higher education and subsequently had careers were displaced. Connie Wilbur was no different. Despite the fact that she was purportedly quite a brilliant psychologist, who could have easily excelled on the higher rungs of psychoanalysis, once the male physicians returned from the war she was pushed aside.

So the timing of her first meeting with Shirley Mason couldn't have been better. Wilbur needed something so intense, so mind-blowing, that the psychoanalytic community would not be able to ignore her. Mason was incredibly feeble and desperate for care. The relationship between the two women (it was a relationship—and not solely a therapeutic one) catapulted them both into the public eye.

We know much about the emotional journey Shirley Mason took with Dr. Wilbur to become Sybil, the years spent recounting the harrowing abuse of her childhood, but much less has been written about her physical ailments, most of which appear to have been written off as a consequence of her hysteria rather than the reverse. An emerging thread seems to be that if a woman is both sick and anxious, she's sick *because* she's anxious—not anxious about being sick. Although much of the work Sybil did psychoanalytically with Wilbur has come under fire in the years following both of their deaths, what one cannot deny is the fairly well-documented medical evidence of Sybil's illness. Early notes on Shirley Mason describe her constellation of physical symptoms—joint aches, fatigue, and debilitating menstrual cramps, from which she had suffered all of her life. In her book *Sybil Exposed*, journalist Debbie Nathan uncovered that at one point during the early years of her treatment, Mason underwent surgery for an ovarian cyst. This same surgery revealed not just a deformed ovary, but endometriosis.

The ovary and endometrial lesions were removed, and reportedly this resolved Mason's menstrual symptoms. For the next few decades of her life, her "nervousness" was treated with heavy barbiturates by her doctors, including Wilbur. Wilbur was particularly fond of sodium pentathol, colloquially referred to as "truth serum," which not only stood to make Sybil more forthcoming, or even suggestible, but presumably could have masked her symptoms with its highly anesthetizing qualities.

Another drug commonly given to women for menstrual symptoms was Daprisal, which Wilbur also readily prescribed. Daprisal was a combination barbiturate painkiller and amphetamine. It disappeared from the market once it was discovered to be highly addictive and easy to overdose on. Trying to find information on it today is next to impossible. One can infer, however, that if Mason was on such an intense cocktail of drugs throughout her reproductive years, her menstrual pain could have conceivably been dulled, or her suffering with them easily forgotten, particularly in the larger context of her struggles. But it is interesting that, yet again, we find a link between a diagnosis of hysteria and the actual physical presence of a painfully diseased reproductive system. It's not a wandering uterus, perhaps—but it isn't one entirely absent of pathology—what you'd called *normal*—either.

PRACTICALLY EVERY ADULT I INTRODUCED myself to once I learned my own name asked me if my parents were Mel Brooks fans, and had I seen *Young Frankenstein* with Gene Wilder? Well, of course I hadn't! I was only five or six years old when these conversations started. Many have observed that my given name reminded them of the famous scene in the film where Marty Feldman's Igor brings a brain to Wilder's Dr. Frankenstein. Whose brain is it?

"Abby someone," Feldman stutters.

"Abby who?" Wilder asks.

"Abby . . . normal."

He had misread the label "Abnormal"—which was not exactly the kind of legacy I was hoping for. So it was, with the kind of fresh, manic self-awareness that only teenagers possess, that my first order of business, after I became legally emancipated from my parents at age sixteen, was to enter therapy. The way I saw it, if I wanted any kind of "normal" adulthood, it would behoove me to start working on my myriad childhood traumas while they were still fresh in my mind, and I was still emotionally malleable enough to overcome them.

For the most part, I was well adjusted in the ways that mattered: I got good grades, had a good reputation, and could hold down a job. I was surviving. I was showing up and doing what I needed to do by the preordained standards of my provincial hometown. But I couldn't shake the feeling that I wasn't exactly *living*. I didn't know if therapy was going to be the solution, but it seemed like a pretty good place to start.

I didn't think I was unsalvageable. I felt that I was very close to self-actualization and, with help, could probably achieve it. I wouldn't say I had hope, but I did lay my faith in the value of hard work. I was willing to confront my demons. What I couldn't have realized as a teenager, however, was that my demons weren't done. I'd approached therapy as salvation, but it turned out to be more like the training for future exorcisms.

There was embarrassingly little thought put into the therapist I would see. One day after school, one of the guidance counselors—the one everyone called by her first name, which was Kim—drove me to the town pier. It was, I'm sure, a peaceful place from her perspective. To me, it was an oasis of memories. My grandmother lived up the street, and I kept looking in the rearview mirror, thinking she'd appear without warning.

The kindly counselor handed me a sheet of paper that had some names on it. therapists in the area who would take Medicaid. The list of names was longer than I would have expected, but I was nervous, so all the letters were blending together. My anxiety about running into my grandmother made my stomach churn. I just wanted to make a decision and leave.

"Would you prefer a female therapist, or would you be open to a man?" Kim asked. *Oh, I'd be open to a man all right*, I thought, thinking the first item on any therapist's checklist for a girl my age would probably be the distinct absence of a boyfriend and the motivation to obtain one.

Finally, I handed the paper back to her and said, "Let's start at the top and work our way down. Just call them and I'll take the first one with an appointment. If I don't like them, we'll try the next one."

She considered this a moment as she squinted at the paper. Then she smiled, reaching for her indestructible little flip-phone. "Jane Jones," she said, tapping the paper with her finger, "I know of her. I bet you'll like her."

I scoffed, wondering if I'd royally goofed. The name Jane Jones sounded so innocuous that I wondered if it was fake. I thought to myself that there must be at least a million Jane Joneses in the world. That it would have been exactly the kind of name I'd use as an alias once I finally moved to New York City and started having dangerous liaisons with mysterious men in ritzy hotel rooms. Perhaps I had spent too much time in school plays, but as far as characters like shrinks went, I would have expected a slightly more interesting name. As it happened, one of a million Jane Joneses could see me the following week.

When I walked into Jane's office in my nicest suit, a manila folder in hand containing all my legal papers, I only had one goal in mind: I wanted to grow up to be normal. I was expecting to sit down and have a very Adult conversation with her. Two Adults talking about Adult things with Adult words in their Adult clothes.

Her office was small, a desk tucked into a far corner, the majority of the room filled with things that a child psychologist would have: a doll's house, books, other toys that were probably meant to act out domestic dramas with. On the wall across from where I lowered myself into a plush, pink wingback chair, there was a painting of a race car, which would ultimately become my preferred focal point.

By way of comparison, dancers have to "spot" their turns—which means finding a focal point that you can very quickly turn your head back to, letting the rest of your body follow. It doesn't completely eliminate the inevitable dizziness, but it helps keep you oriented to the space. That painting was how I spotted in therapy. When the space would spin and cave in on itself, it was how I found my way back.

I looked unabashedly around the room. It was my nature to take in my surroundings quickly, a tendency I assume I developed as a survival instinct. I memorized every detail of her office in just a few minutes, and years later I can still see it: the way the sun came in through the sheer blinds next to me, the knitted cover of the rocking chair that neither of us ever sat in, the diplomas on the wall behind her desk, and the books on her shelves.

And, of course, Jane herself.

Somehow I'd expected her to be wearing a suit as well, but she was not. I guessed she was in her late forties. She was petite, and pretty in the way your best friend's mom is pretty. There was a softness about her blonde, blue-eyed mien. Her voice had a balmy, melodic, almost hypnotic quality to it, which is something that I often wondered about. Did therapists get trained to sound that way, or do people who naturally sound like that just end up in social work?

This first meeting was the first of many in which I was over-dressed for the occasion. It was summer, and Jane, while still manag-ing to present an air of consummate professionalism, sat across from me in her office barefoot. I don't remember exactly what she wore that first day, but over the years she'd rotate through a never-ending wardrobe of sundresses and jumpers, with the occasional pastel car-digan thrown in. She either wore no makeup at all, or wore so little that it was barely perceptible—which I found rather impressive. It had never really occurred to me before that cosmetics might be op-tional. I'd been begrudgingly putting my face on every day since I was around fourteen.

I noticed fairly quickly that she wasn't wearing a wedding ring, which was something that, at that age, I always noticed about peo-ple, despite having no reason to interpret its presence or absence other than to indulge my own burgeoning curiosity about adulthood. My immediate assumption was that she was divorced. She was self-possessed in a way that made her seem unattached, like she wasn't itching to be somewhere else. People who are intensely coupled al-ways seem to me to have a certain energy; it's as though they're being pulled elsewhere—as if they are forever trying to get back to their other half.

I likewise assumed she was childless, as I picked up no maternal vibe from her whatsoever. It might sound strange, but this was actu-ally a great relief to me. Women sometimes looked at me with a cer-tain kind of feminine pity that made me squirm. But I'd only just met Jane; there was still time for her to give me Sad Mom Eyes.

Having reached the conclusion that she wasn't a mother, I imme-diately decided I liked her. Never one to enter a situation unarmed, I had read up on what therapy would be like and, upon coming across the term *transference*, had balked at the idea that I would develop misplaced emotional attachment to some middle-aged woman I was paying to listen to me gripe. My understanding of human relation-ships (and the foundational principles of psychoanalytic theory, as it were) at age sixteen was founded in dysfunction and inexperience. Therefore every relationship, manufactured or not, I expected to be dysfunctional.

With that in mind, I was anxious to create some kind of emotionally unavailable life for Jane. It made her seem less threatening. The thing about therapy is that the entire relationship is built on having only half-truths about your therapist, while the therapist gets to know you intimately. I thought it sounded, in theory, like the strangest relationship two humans could undertake. I was going to be telling her things I'd never told anyone else. I was going to end up vulnerable, which was frightening. I created a sort of featureless life for her in my mind to both humanize and dehumanize her. I was all at once desperate for her to see me and to bear witness to what I had to tell her, and terrified that she would see something more than what I decided to give. I felt the need to make her less threatening, somehow, because I didn't want to imagine her going home at night to tut about my Tragic Backstory while her husband rubbed her feet and brought her another glass of merlot.

Although my brain couldn't help but spin its wheels to sum Jane up, I also felt like the early misconceptions I adopted about her were more about distancing myself from the real emotional work I knew would be necessary. By creating this life for her—which, I would find out later, couldn't have been more wrong—I was attempting to make her safe. I was trying to fortify myself so that I wouldn't just get up and run out the second it got hard. I wanted therapy to work. I wanted to change.

The first thing Jane did that day was lean over the low, glass-topped table that stood between us so that she could inspect my emancipation paperwork. She stared at it for what seemed like forever, and I cavalierly crossed my legs, looking down the bridge of my nose at her. The moment burned out slowly, like a cigarette, and I swallowed back the ache of melancholy as it bloomed in my throat.

"If you have any concerns about their validity, you can contact my attorney," I announced blithely, stretching my fingers out long so that I could pretend to be entertained by my well-trimmed fingernails.

She shrugged, setting the paperwork down on the table and looking at me with a sort of benevolent amusement.

"I don't question their validity at all," she said evenly. "I only asked you to bring them out of curiosity." She tipped her head slightly, settling back into her wingback chair as her gaze settled onto me. "I've never seen emancipation papers before."

Over the first few months, I saw Jane weekly after school, dutifully regaling her with my tale of woe. Starting, I suppose, with all the pain that had come before me; that I had come from. Starting—with an all-too Freudian aplomb—with my mother.

—⁂—

SHE WAS ALWAYS *MUM*—NEVER MOM, never Mama, never Mommy. When my life began, she was living with my father in a trailer park near where he worked as a lineman for the power company. Thus, all my childhood memories of my father involve steel-toed boots, the scent of diesel fuel, and that particular brand of working-class masculinity that includes metal lockers adorned with swimsuit models and break rooms full of finicky soda machines.

Dad's job was not a cushy one. Maine winters can be unforgiving. During The ice Storm of '98, I came to understand just how hard my father worked. He was gone for months cleaning up the aftermath of that storm. The entire state became a desolate, frozen hellhole. There was no school. People had lost power, and many of them, in the now arctic northeast, had no running water. Dad and his crew set out to clear downed trees that groaned and snapped under sheets of solid ice, and to restore power to thousands of households along the East Coast. He and his crew climbed telephone poles in subzero temperatures, worked long hours that would probably be illegal by today's standards, and slept in their trucks. They relied on the kindness of strangers for warm meals and encouragement.

When he finally came home, he seemed to have aged about ten years. He was in his early thirties at the time, but I'm pretty sure that storm took a few years off the lives of everyone who lived through it. I understood, then, what it meant to have a good work ethic. Dad was often called into work in the middle of the night during storms, worked endless hours of overtime doing backbreaking and, in fact, dangerous work. Yet I can count on one hand the number of times he called in sick—and when he did, he always really *was* sick. Or, in the later years, taking care of my mother when she was.

Dad never said any of this to me. He was, and remains, a man of few words. Most of my childhood memories of him are from the side—looking at him in profile as he watched television or stood in front of the bathroom mirror to shave. My fondest memories of him are riding in the front seat of his old white pickup listening to The Brian Setzer Orchestra, willing him to look up and see me.

Of my parents, it was my mother who saw me, although I spent the better part of my childhood wishing she couldn't. From the moment I implanted into my mother's womb, I became a statistically improbable event. Mum had been told that because she was at such low weight, she wouldn't be able to get pregnant—yet I manifested. I was an unlikely child, sure, but did that mean I was inherently unlovable?

Mum, at barely twenty-four and extremely ill, was in no position to care for, let alone love, a baby. To add insult to injury, my beginning was not auspicious: the first thing I did as a human infant was shit all over the place. Poor Mum lay semiconscious from hemorrhaging while I exercised my newfound lung capacity and began a lifetime of questionable bowel function.

Apparently, I cried inconsolably for the first few months of my life, and eventually went on to become insufferable in other ways that grated on Mum's already fragile nerves. She coped the only way she knew how: she vomited. *A lot.*

Anorexia and bulimia often occur together in a cringe-worthy symbiosis. Mum started out restricting her food when she was just a preteen. Her grandmother, who had been her only solace, had died, and it sent Mum into a massive clinical depression. One that, unfortunately, went unnoticed and untreated—in large part because her mother, my grandmother, had untreated mental illness as well.

Mum's life was an unfortunate, but not uncommon, perfect storm: my grandmother was a poor, working, single mother with untreated mental illness and limited social support. It's a tale as old as time. Rural, small-town neighborhoods are often enablers of abusive homes. The one Mum grew up in was no exception, and all her life she's remained bitter that no one—no neighbor, no teacher, no family friend—ever stepped in to help her.

My mother's struggles really solidified when she was in high school in the 1980s, about four years after she had begun restricting her food intake. At the time, bulimia was becoming somewhat fashionable. A few girls in her class had "tried it out," and a few weeks of purging later, the scratchy throats, bloodshot eyes, and uncomfortable hunger were enough to turn them off from it.

Mum, however, had found it rather soothing; it provided the comfort she'd been seeking since her grandmother's death. Purging gave her a sleepy, contented feeling that mitigated the anxiety and fear at home. It was never about weight: the dopamine-producing binge-and-purge sessions rendered her environment, and herself, tolerable, her life survivable.

When she married my father in her early twenties, she'd already had an eating disorder for nearly a decade. It wasn't that he didn't know about her bulimia, he just didn't understand the significance of it. In his defense, in the late 1980s and early 1990s there were few people who did. This was thirty-some years ago, when these things weren't discussed on daytime talk shows. There were no "pro-ana" websites or Dr. Phil specials. I don't think my father really understood what she was doing. Her family knew, and had known, but they were ashamed of it, and disgusted. Getting her help wasn't necessarily their first priority—keeping her "filthy habit" a secret was.

As the challenges of growing up gripped her psyche, her weight quickly began to plummet. When she was twenty three years old, just before she got pregnant with me, she was five-foot-five and weighed less than one hundred pounds.

By the time my brother was born a year and a half later, from the beginning something wasn't quite right. Then again, Mum had hardly been healthy during her pregnancy. She'd been running after a toddler—me—and hadn't exactly recovered from her eating disorder. If anything, motherhood had made the bulimia more of a necessity than before.

As a little girl, especially after my brother was born, I spent a lot of time with Mum's mother, who I called Nana. When I was very young my relationship with her was a good one: she took me to flea markets, we baked cookies, and puttered around in the garden. She lived a short walk from the bay, and I could play on the shore with the neighborhood kids until dark. I came to prefer being at her house over being at home for these reasons, though as I got older the dynamic began to shift. In the same way I would eventually come to understand that my mother's treatment wasn't based in hatred, I don't think Nana's mistreatment of her, and eventually of me as well, was about hate either. My mother was deeply afraid that she would repeat the same abusive patterns with her children that her mother had subjected her and her siblings to. Although my mother was beaten repeatedly throughout her childhood (and, on a few occasions, even after she had grown up, moved out, and gotten married), she never beat me or my brother.

In that way, if not others, she had broken the cycle. Though sadly, as I grew up, I'd come to realize that one reason she had so little to offer me was that she had never truly been able to escape the unhealthy dynamic she had with her own mother. Everything in her life, including herself—including me—was viewed through that warped lens.

Consequently, I learned the word "manipulation" fairly early in life, having existed in a disordered triangulation between my mother and grandmother. I figured out many years too late that I was a pawn in their dysfunctional relationship. It was, at times, almost like being in the middle of two bitterly divorced parents: whenever I was with one of them, they spent a lot of time and energy disparaging and undermining the other. It seemed I existed only to make them miserable—that is to say, I was used by both of them to make *each other* miserable.

As I began to grow—my body shooting up closer to the sky, chest punctuated with painful breast buds that I despised, hair on my legs that seemed darker than any hair I'd ever seen on my head—my mother's resentment of me became more personal. At least, that's how it felt to me at that age. I understand now that it was all to do with *her*, and she more than likely didn't hate me. She hated herself so much she didn't have the energy to hate—or love—anyone else.

One thing I found jarring in those years was that both my mother and my grandmother seemed to lack certain boundaries. It was almost as though my body was just an extension of them, and that they needed to be in control of it. One example of this being that Mum insisted on washing my hair until I was into my preteen years, which she justified by saying that I couldn't do it well enough myself. That may very well have been true, because I had never been taught.

Even as a child, I thought that she was exacting more control over me than was strictly necessary, and that if she felt that I was doing things incorrectly, then, as the parent, the solution should be to teach me to do them properly—rather than enforcing learned helplessness. Mum always maintained that I "never needed her" as a child, though what I recall of my childhood with her makes me suspect that she, in some way, came to need me.

She exacted much control over my appearance, even rouging my cheeks when I was in elementary school—I imagine so that I wouldn't look so pale. My pallor being evidence of the other area in which she dictated every decision: food. I wasn't allowed to eat unless she specifically gave me a pre-portioned snack or meal. I was hungry most of the day, and soon got into the habit of stealing food at school, which I subsequently started to hoard.

While I had been gaining inches and experience, she had been getting smaller, as had her world. Sometimes she'd be slumped on the scratchy living-room carpet, and she'd ask me to come rub her back. I would cower, turning my head as I lifted up her nightdress. I could count each of her ribs; they protruded so severely that I thought they'd rip straight through her skin. If she moved, even slightly, I could see the outline of her internal organs, which pulsated slowly, almost as though they were grinding up against one another. Her once pretty jet black hair had thinned, and she wore it cropped close to her skull. Her face, if she would turn it up to look at me (which she rarely did), was hollowed out, her eyes sunk so far back into her skull that they were nothing but shadows, like cut-out eyes in a mask. Her lips were dry and cracked, caked with blood or vomit in the corners. She was pale, her skin papery thin and translucent. She was always freezing cold, and the bones of her hands, joints, and knees stuck out at strange angles.

During these years, I had a recurring nightmare of a skeleton chasing me, its bony fingers curling, reaching for me—begging me to help them find their skin.

Although she faltered, as all mothers do, one thing Mum imparted to me, that I give credit to her unequivocally and with deep appreciation, was a love of books. The only memories I have of her that are not besmirched by food, or anger, or purgatives, are those of her reading. She read all the time, every day, unceasingly. Before she became gravely ill, she could easily read a few books a week. She read voraciously, and she read everything: the more obvious choices, like cookbooks and self-help, but there were always dog-eared biographies of queens and contemporary fiction about. There were books everywhere, all around her, around us. I was very fortunate that books were so highly accessible to me so early in life.

While Mum may have denied me some food and some love, she never denied me a book. It didn't matter what the topic was, who the author was, or even how much it cost. She would never say no to a book. Even when I was in the fifth grade and developed an inexhaustible fascination with the Kennedy family, deciding I wanted to read every biography that had ever been written on every member of the clan (of which there are many, many, many). At one point I came across a gorgeous coffee-table book of all the gowns that had been designed for Jackie, mostly by Oleg Cassini. The book cost $50.00 and it wasn't a book that most people would sit down and read cover to cover—but I would. And my mother knew that, so she bought it for me. Fifteen years later, I still have it on my bookshelf.

It was around this time, or maybe a bit before, that the family pediatrician deemed me "precocious"—which, in spite of our mutual love of books, was really the last breed of child Mum wanted to deal with. Namely, because her entire existence was based on secrecy, the success of which depended on the stupidity, self-absorption, and obliviousness of those around her.

I didn't believe for one second that the hours she spent behind the closed bathroom door were spent "brushing her teeth." Yes, there was some tooth-brushing involved in the end (evidenced by the occasional sour taste on the bristles of my toothbrush), but I knew she was up to something else entirely. I couldn't prove it, but I also wasn't sure I wanted to know the truth.

We lived in a thin-walled, double-wide trailer, and they don't accommodate secret-keeping. It was always dark, no matter the time of day, because there were blankets draped over the windows. A heavy layer of dust covered everything, because nothing was ever touched or moved from its resting place; it was a museum of unheld things. The whir of fans running year-round kept it chilled like a tomb. It was its own kind of bizarre sensory deprivation; time and place, day and night, were simply lost to me in those years.

From the outside, it didn't look much different from any other weather-worn Maine house: crooked and derelict. A set of rickety stairs, painted pale blue, chipped away after years of neglect, was balanced somewhat haphazardly against the door. There was a gap between the siding and the top step, and as soon as I stepped onto it from the trailer, it would give beneath me, the whole staircase wobbling a bit to the side. I'd reach for the splintered railing, the bright sun disorienting. Leaving the house was always like waking up from a bad dream.

In photographs I often appear worn and tired, dark circles under my eyes. I was a dervish in a doll's house: pale, porcelain skin, thin in the way a little girl shouldn't be. But I'm almost always smiling, sometimes painfully so. My hair was a mousy brown and very fine, which meant it erred on the side of greasy. I wore crookedly cut bangs across my forehead, the rest of it dusting my shoulders, and later (and for most of my life thereafter) in an impish, chin-length bob. I harbored fantasies about someone brushing it for me.

I was alone so much that one morning, when I was probably around seven or eight, I woke up and decided I must be a ghost. It seemed plausible: no one could apparently see me or hear me, and I was slowly losing my ability to feel things (like emotions and hunger pains).

I was a proficient haunt by the age of ten, a clandestine child biting the inside of her cheek until it went raw. Pain meant I was corporeal, but I kept my humanness cleverly concealed by porcelain baby teeth and chapped lips, as if not to trouble anyone else with it.

I used to sit in my father's closet, tucked away behind his golf clubs, torn shoe boxes, and sweaters I'd never seen him wear, with my back pressed up against the wall. On the other side, the washer and dryer would run at least a few times a day, and their humming became a mechanical comfort. I would close my eyes and let the warmth of the vents soothe me, the gentle *ka-thump* . . . *ka-thump* . . . *ka-thump* of the dryer cycle like a heartbeat against my fledgling human form. I daydreamed of a soft-spoken lady, aglow like the angels in Sunday school, opening the door and her arms to me. Then, the dryer would stop, and I would grow cold. At first, I would reach up to gently stroke the sleeve of my father's unworn sweaters, but I would later discover that I was allergic to wool.

I was not a ghost. I was a little girl with needs and wants and allergies. Still, I hung soundlessly, as weightlessly as I could, in the air. The living can haunt a house, too.

All the doors in the trailer were made of some kind of plywood, with a plasticky, Barbie-House-style, lacquered finish that gave them a rather wimpy appearance. I spent a large part of my childhood with my back up against those doors, my ear pressed against the cool surfaces. What I'm saying is, I know my modular home doors.

These memories, like many things that later prove fatal, start with a cough.

It was a hollow sound my mother made. I thought she must practically have her head in the sink because of how it echoed. Acoustics were the first clue. Time would pass while I sat outside the bathroom door, wearing down the carpet trying to figure out if I was a girl or a ghost. She would emerge, bleary-eyed and hoarse, and snap at me upon realizing I'd been sitting there listening.

At the time, I took it personally, as little children do. I would slip inside the bathroom in her wake and immediately be pummeled with the sickly, sour smell that I knew, but couldn't quite place. A smell invariably mixed with the homespun scent of Lysol. Occasionally, it would be laced with lavender soap, a feeble spritz in an attempt to hide the stench.

Over the years, we all became scent-blind to the smell of stagnant vomit. I became deaf to the sound of her retching. Like the whir of a box fan or the cyclical thud of the dryer, it was just the din of my home.

These sights, sounds, and smells were frequently interlaced with those of my brother's tantrums, which years later we'd find out were a hallmark of autism. When he was little, they almost always culminated with literal shit-slinging. He wasn't potty trained for an inordinately long time, and when he was frustrated, lacking the proper communication skills, more often than not, he'd wipe feces on the walls or grind it into the rugs. I used to sit in the middle of the living-room floor and pretend the bleach spots in the carpet were islands for my Barbies to lounge on.

Mum was exhausted from her constant cycle of bingeing and purging, but my brother's harrowing tantrums would have been enough to fray the nerves of someone far better adjusted than she was.

I was ten when Andrea Yates drowned her children in the bathtub, and I remember the news coverage quite vividly. Newscasters didn't mince words about what she had done, and I'm sure most kids that age can comprehend what killing is. I don't suppose, however, that most children would have understood how such a thing could have happened. Yates was a fragile, dark-haired, somber-looking woman, like Mum. Whenever they showed her image on TV, I would stare unflinchingly at her—the way I had never dared to look at my own mother.

As the broadcasts droned on in the living room, I remember standing in the hallway, once again on the other side of that closed bathroom door, wondering if Mum ever thought about drowning us. A fear flitted through me. Not because I thought she might—but because some nights, I wished that she would.

The only control my mother had—or believed she had—was the command she had over food. As a child, I interpreted her restriction of my food as cruelty. As hatred. But as I've gotten older and have come to understand the psychology, and physiology, of eating disorders, I see that for her, there was no other choice.

That being said, whatever her intentions may have been, the fact remains that I spent a large part of my childhood hungry. Really hungry. I would come home from school and have eaten my dinner—my last supper—by four o'clock in the afternoon. My father usually was home from work by five, at which time Mum disappeared into her bedroom, not to be seen again until the following morning. I would sometimes watch my father eat, which unsettled him deeply. I'd sit there, wordlessly staring at whatever he was eating, trying to imagine that I was eating it too. Mum generally only let me eat very specific things, and in very small portions. I remember seeing a great deal of skinless chicken breast, bland almost to the point of being sterile, on equally colorless plates, or slightly withered patties of ground beef that seemed oddly vulnerable in the absence of a bun.

By the time the sun had gone down and my father was staring blankly at the TV, I'd tiptoe into the kitchen to forage. Dad was in the next room—a living room that might as well have been in the middle of the kitchen, given the narrow length of the trailer we lived in—but he was far away. I would move silently, methodically, having planned out my moves like a highly trained operative. I'd envision my success several times before I put my plan in motion: I calculated how many steps from my bedroom to the kitchen, tried to map out how to move a kitchen chair, soundlessly, and place it in front of the counter so I could reach the cabinets. Sometimes, if moving a chair felt too risky, I'd just throw a leg over the edge of the sink and yank my little body up until it came down with a thump against the countertops with some impressive parkour. As I struggled to maintain my balance, I would duck and open the green cabinet door, quickly scanning the contents. I was looking for something quick, easy, and quiet that would hold me over until morning.

Dad would sit motionless in his chair watching television while I moved like a thief in the night, feeling like I was robbing my own house.

Sometimes I was successful. I would retreat to my room with a handful or two of pretzels in the dip of my nightdress, which I would yank up in front of me like a little food hammock, a pouch. But sometimes, I wouldn't succeed. Sometimes Mum would hear me, and she'd come stomping out of her dark cave, half-asleep and angry. If I heard her open the door, I'd scamper down off the counter and into my room like a feral animal, maybe a pretzel or two crammed in my mouth. But if she moved soundlessly, and snuck up on me like a predator on her prey, then the bark of her voice from the dark would send me crashing down onto the floor, having toppled from the counter empty-handed, breathless, scared. A few times, the edge of the sink caught my leg or my arm, painfully wrenching it, nearly dislodging it from its hip or shoulder socket. We would stare each other down before retreating back into the night, both of us empty, hungry, and alone.

The next morning I would wake up for school and revel in those blissful few moments before my body was fully awake, numb to hunger and shame. Mum would already be puking in the bathroom next to my room, trying to achieve the same effect.

Hunger was more difficult to ignore at school because it often interfered with my ability to concentrate. On the other hand, school was the better place to be because it was easier to get snacks. I was the queen of "Are you going to eat that?" by the time I reached the third grade. I subsisted on other people's scraps, which would have horrified my mother, had she caught me—obviously, because it was food, but also because I was exposing myself to germs. If there was one thing that troubled Mum more than food, it was illness—especially the vomiting variety.

It might seem odd, since vomiting was her whole life—but seeing or hearing someone else do it was enormously triggering for her, since she was so profoundly bulimic. It had, by proxy, become enormously triggering for me, too. I just didn't understand what, exactly, I was afraid of.

All I know is that I can tell you every single time I vomited as a child. On every occasion, I was terrified and she was angry, disgusted, and dismissive. I didn't grasp that she felt that way about herself, not me. Her transference of misplaced blame was too much nuance for me, especially when I was sick in the middle of the night.

Fearing this, whenever I begged for other kids' snacks, my heart would thump away wildly in my chest. Is it worth it to eat this if it makes me sick? Is it better to go hungry than get germs on me? I would weigh these options every single time, so much so that it became something of a mantra. Some days, the fear of getting sick and making Mum angry was too great, so I wouldn't eat. Some days, the hunger won. As I got older and tried to grow, the hunger won a lot more. Still, during the months of the year when influenza circulated, I would become paralyzed with fear, therefore not eating enough, and would wind up in the nurse's station. I wouldn't be able to see the chalkboard, or I'd start shaking from low blood sugar, slumping onto the floor, or not be able to play at recess. I'd lie on a scratchy cot in the nurse's office and cry.

By the time elementary school came to an end, I still wasn't sure what I was supposed to fear more: what would happen if I ate, or what would happen if I didn't.

When I got sick, cruelly, one of the first and most persistent symptoms I had was intractable nausea. Regardless of whatever food was in front of me, I couldn't have more than a few bites. To compound the issue, I wasn't sleeping well. I had always been an early-to-bed, early-to-rise kind of girl. At college, I'd only pulled an all-nighter once, and really, it hadn't been a true all-nighter, because I was in bed before 4 a.m. But now, the pain and nausea, combined with my mounting anxiety, kept me awake all night, every night, for about six weeks. I was so sleep- and nutrient-deprived that I remember very little about that period of my life. Luckily, I journaled constantly. The journal entries reflect the chaos of that time, the overwhelming sadness and confusion, the pain—and the preoccupations.

One thing that happened almost immediately was that I became fearful I was developing an eating disorder like my mother. Even though I wanted to eat, and it seemed to be something mechanical that was causing my stomach to reject my efforts, I thought about my mother all the time. I wondered if all of this was my subconscious trying to make me anorexic, or, worse yet, bulimic.

Although I had downright feared vomiting as a child, by the time I entered college, and even toward the end of high school, I had the distinct displeasure of cleaning up after drunken pals, and I became a bit desensitized. I was still apprehensive about getting sick on a somewhat visceral level that I couldn't quite explain. It felt as though my body was afraid of something that my mind hadn't yet been made aware of, and at so much as the mention of a stomach virus circulating, or the potential of food poisoning, I felt an inexplicable panic that couldn't be quelled. I tried to explain to myself that it was just holdover from my childhood, a kind of *vomitrocious* posttraumatic stress. It wasn't until I was nearly out of high school that I had an experience that contextualized that fear.

On the surface, it's not a very interesting story: I threw up at the Olive Garden. I don't know why. I was fine beforehand, and then, quite suddenly, broke out into a cold sweat and leapt up from the table, dashing off toward the bathroom, having not yet had the opportunity to stuff any breadsticks into my purse. There was a moment of panic at the realization that I was about to vomit, mostly because it occurred to me that I hadn't done so in a long time, and maybe I wouldn't remember what to do.

Of course, it being an autonomic function, more or less, I didn't really have to do anything. It just happened. But when it did, in that long moment that followed, something peculiar came over me. At first I thought it was relief—though I hadn't even been nauseated beforehand, which is usually why people find vomiting to be so alleviating. No, it wasn't relief. It was a kind of giddiness. I was flushed from head to toe in a deep, resonant calm. All the tension had melted from my body—tension that I hadn't even realized had existed, except that I noted its absence. I had not realized that I could take such deep breaths, or that my fingers could be so soft and unfurled. I was a bit lightheaded, but not dizzy. I felt emptied of more than overpriced pasta—it was almost as though I'd had some kind of spiritual experience, an exorcism when I hadn't even known I'd been possessed.

To be perfectly blunt, I felt high as fuck. I'd never done any "hard drugs," but I'd smoked a little reefer in my day. I'd watched other people get high a lot, though, as I was often the token sober friend, the mom, the designated driver. Bongs made out of Arizona iced tea cans, technicolor tabs of acid that had cartoons on them like cereal box prizes, lines of coke on water-damaged manga you read from back to front. I knew what people looked like when they were high. I also knew what addiction looked like.

I leaned against the wall of the bathroom stall, letting my eyes close. There was a hesitant knock on the door, and someone asked if I was all right. I laughed in the affirmative. I felt fucking great. I flushed the toilet with my foot and stepped out of the stall to wash my hands. When I looked into the mirror over the sink, I stopped short.

My eyes were too wide, too alight, wild and dark. My face was flushed and I was smiling almost manically, showing all my teeth. I marveled at how much air I was breathing, how everything around me appeared brighter and anew. I returned to the table and to my friend, who had been worried. I took a swig of water and grabbed my purse, practically skipping out of the restaurant. She offered to drive, even though she technically didn't have her license, because she was worried I was too ill.

I told her I wasn't ill, that I felt fine. Amazing, in fact. I started the car, and it wasn't until I put my hands on the wheel that I realized I was shaking, vibrating almost. I was energized, thoroughly charged. I amped the radio and drove too fast to get home.

The comedown came later, and I didn't realize it was even happening at first. I just felt sleepy, overtired. Then my nerves crackled under my skin, snapping and popping. I stood in the bathroom and thought, for one grotesque moment, how delightful it would feel to let my skin slough off my bones, falling to the floor like a damp towel.

It hit me fast and hard—a sickening, terrifying realization, a mental nausea stilling me so that my hand had to shoot out to balance me against the wall, lest I fall. I wanted to throw up again. I wanted to throw up, because I wanted that feeling. I knew, instinctively, that I would feel that way, that I would get my reward. I knew that was why my mother had done it. The cycle of addiction, children of addicts becoming addicts. That's why I'd only watched with vague fascination as my friends did drugs. Why I only pretended to drink, dumping a friend's mother's cheap boxed wine into a nearby potted plant. That's why even when I was no longer afraid of disappointing my mother, I had scrubbed my hands until they were raw, because I knew it would only take one heave, one time, one single puke— .

The disgust that I had come to feel toward my mother as a teenager was suddenly turned full force upon myself. I did not throw up that night. In fact, several more years would elapse, during which time my efforts to prevent it were motivated by a secret fear that I did not share with anyone, because I found it humiliating.

Then, my first year at Sarah Lawrence, it happened again. I don't remember exactly what preceded it. I'd probably been up too late having too much coffee. I think I'd eaten a strange concoction of crispy, undercooked Ramen and fuzzy candy I'd dug out from the bottom of my messenger bag. I tried, earnestly, not to vomit. Soon, though, I realized that I was wasting time—precious time that I needed to work and, God willing, to sleep. It was over in half a second, and there wasn't even much to show for it. But immediately I was flooded by that feeling that couldn't be matched, that I hadn't forgotten but had been too afraid to chase. Unlike when I'd had the peculiar experience in high school, by the time I was in college I'd smoked rich-kid marijuana and taught myself how to orgasm. So when I felt my knees buckle under the weight of that serene ecstasy, I knew just how good it really was. So, too, I understood how dangerous it was, how potentially fatal.

I sat in the bathroom with my back pressed up against the cabinet beneath the bathroom sink. Several weeks earlier, I'd dropped a cherished earring down the drain. At first I panicked, until I remembered that I'd brought along a toolkit that was living in my closet, still in plastic. I calmly laid out the wrench, the pliers, a small auger.

I threw down some towels, grabbed a big bowl from the kitchen to stick under the sink, and rolled up my sleeves. It was a problem that I had everything I needed to solve. The distress I'd felt watching the tiny amethyst disappear into the dark was replaced by a sense of assurance. I knew I would be able to retrieve it if I focused and employed a bit of elbow-grease. Sometime later, I shimmied out from beneath the sink, the tiny jewel shimmering in my damp palm. I smiled, pleased with myself for being able to avert a crisis without having to ask for help.

Leaning up against that sink weeks later, I realized that being good in a crisis required more than a passing knowledge of plumbing, and that there were some catastrophes that couldn't be handled alone. I went back to bed and lay awake for the rest of the night, convincing myself that I had enough self-control to keep myself from getting sick again. I thought that having thrown up was the crisis, but the real danger lay in the fact that I knew, as I fell asleep, that I would wake up in the morning and want, desperately, to do it again.

Years later, I'd lay awake in bed all night, too exhausted to sleep. The first six months after I got sick, those fears of inevitable bulimia and anorexia came back to me. The nausea that had started at Sarah Lawrence had not left me, and after months of not eating much, it had turned into a vicious cycle: eventually, the not-eating nauseated me just as much as trying to eat. No matter what I did, my guts were in a constant state of churning that often got so severe it stole my breath. I knew I had to find something I could tolerate, because I was losing too much weight, and too fast. My attempts to investigate food and find something that worked preoccupied me so much that I began to display the very kind of eating-disordered behaviors that my mother had.

Eventually, I found certain things that I could tolerate: saltines, dried cranberries, clear soups. But I became terrified of everything else. I spent an inordinate amount of time Googling pictures of all the foods that I couldn't eat anymore, and stared pathetically at them at 1 a.m. when I was wide awake from malnourishment, pain, and the fear that all of this was some kind of prophecy—self-fulfilling or otherwise. I soon figured out that not-eating gave me a similarly calm, high feeling. It wasn't as full-bodied or delicious as the one that I got when I threw up, but it was the only feeling, besides pain, that my body seemed to be able to generate. I fought against it, plied my body with nutrition—only to be so nauseated, as my body attempted to digest even small amounts of food, that I would once again be saddled by the feeling of impending doom.

Things were different now in a terrifying way: before when I had thrown up, I had not been depressed. I'd had other things to focus on, and abounding happiness in most areas of my life that gave me the resolve I needed to avoid descending into an addiction I could see I was at risk for developing. But when all of that was taken from me, and my days became an endless slog of strange, elongated hours of pain endured in darkened rooms, I would close my eyes against the spinning world and give myself a simple, but sobering, warning: If you throw up now, you'll never stop.

WHEN I WAS ABOUT TWELVE years old, Mum almost died. Her weight had plummeted—she weighed about the average for an eight-year-old girl. Not surprisingly, she had become nearly comatose from malnutrition and was actively dying. I sat in the back seat as Nana drove us a few hours south to commit Mum to a hospital.

Her illness was my first experience with doctors shrugging and scratching their heads a lot. Many of them lacked compassion for her, which frustrated me. I felt entitled to hate her, but where did they get off being so curiously unfeeling? I was under the impression that doctors were there to heal patients, not that patients existed so doctors could practice medicine.

There wasn't much left to Mum by this point—physically or otherwise. We were both sitting in the back seat of my grandmother's Taurus, and I watched as she struggled to find whatever remaining vim she had to protest. At one point during her requiem, I became uncharacteristically piqued. I announced, with exactly as much tact as you'd expect a preteen girl to have, that I was hoping she'd die so we could all move on with our lives. In response, she summoned the vestiges of her strength and slapped me hard across the face.

When she was admitted, I went to live with Nana, and although I was only twelve years old, I would never live with my parents again.

At the time, I didn't know that, and so I went to school the next day
as if nothing were wrong. I casually informed my few close friends
that it seemed my mother was finally dying—like, for real this time.
They all had recognized on some level that she was a little off: she
made a point of policing the food at birthday parties, for example,
and she'd never been to one of my school plays. Although they didn't
know much about her, my pals seemed jarred by the news of her impending death. I suppose it really wasn't so surprising. On the outside, it must have appeared quite simple: all they needed to know was
that she was my mother, and that she was probably dying. At the very
least, my calm and collected attitude about it must have unnerved
them. The adults in my life, namely teachers, were none the wiser,
as far as I could tell. I was my same old pedantic, weird self—dying
mom or no.

The first time I intentionally reached out for scraps of love in a
classroom setting was in the first grade. I had a soft-spoken, wool-
sweater-clad teacher named Mrs. Neman. She had an airy halo of
walnut hair and bright, kind eyes that always looked happy to see us.
She read us *Charlotte's Web* in her soft little lamb's voice and assured
me there was no reason girls couldn't get excited about dinosaurs.

Mrs. Neman was perhaps the first person to notice my aptitude
for language. She encouraged all of us to write our own stories, but
I remember that she seemed particularly proud of me. Maybe she
wasn't. But since I'd never felt that someone was proud of me before,
it felt magnanimous to me. I marveled every day that she paid me any
attention at all. I was so overwhelmed every time she wrote "Wonderful!" in her pretty script at the top of my stories that it would make
me cry. I still have a few of them, salvaged from moves and water
damage and anger. In recent years, as an adult, I started looking back
at them, reliving the stories I was really telling at the age of six and
seven. They were quite revealing.

There were bad little children stealing food and being sent to
their rooms. Mean mothers with angry inverted triangle eyebrows.
What gutted me the most was a story about a family of mice in which
I wrote they were "a very nice family—but baby was awful."

Awful seems like such a strong and specific word for a little child to use, particularly when it seems to be something of an

autobiographical statement. I've since been informed that in play therapy, children who have not yet acquired the kind of language that would permit them to put their experiences into words often repeat the same themes over and over again in their imaginative play. This is probably why the other kids stopped asking me to play house— unless I was the dad, in which case I left soon after the game began and went into a corner to read my book until "dinner" was served.

I guess I've been using storytelling to try to understand myself since childhood. Thanks to that first-grade teacher who thought my stories were wonderful, I became confident in my storytelling ability. I guess I just spent the rest of my young life hoping someone would think that I was wonderful even if I didn't have a story to tell.

Many years after my baby-mice stories had long disappeared to collect dust in an old shoebox, there would be a person like that in my life: a vivacious and steadfast woman named Cass.

Once you arrived in middle school, you were informed posthaste that Mrs. Cassandra McCue, science teacher extraordinaire, was essentially everyone's favorite teacher. Therefore, the competition for her affections was stiff.

As it is for many, middle school was a strange time for me. Most of the girls my age were bopping around in their hip-hugger jeans and writing Savage Garden lyrics in their notebooks with glitter gel pens. My wardrobe was entirely made up of a contrarian mix of black business suits and flea-market finery that made me look about twice my age. The only hint that I wasn't an adult was that only rarely did these items of clothing end up on a proper hanger. Forgoing gel pens for black Pilots, I lined the margins of my notebooks with plot diagrams for *X-Files* fan fiction.

Mrs. McCue took a liking to me at first because of my rather unique fashion sense. She still recalls, some fifteen years later, a pastel yellow trench coat the color of an Easter basket that I wore with aplomb. I imagine she thought a little positive attention from her, as opposed to being mercilessly teased by my peers, might help me socially.

I laugh today about my penchant for wearing vintage dresses, many of which were God-awful hand-me-downs from friends of Nana, or yard-sale finds. I was quite ahead of my time in terms of hipster trends, I guess. I even had a very respectable collection of silk scarves, which I wore daily—another affinity I shared with Mrs. McCue.

The year before we started high school, it was announced that she would be reassigned, therefore moving up with us to teach ninth grade. Everyone was thrilled, but for me it was also a relief, because I'd taken to confiding in Mrs. McCue (who became just "Cass" to me after school when I'd hang around), about my problems at home.

Cass, meanwhile, didn't seem to have quite so many problems. She was in her late forties, well-dressed, with coiffed, caramel-highlighted chestnut hair. Like me, she wore high heels every day, and my classmates said that when they heard the clacking down the hallway, they could never tell which one of us it was. Also like me, she had a carefully constructed wardrobe, though unlike me, she had an enviable jewelry collection as well, and she always smelled of Chanel perfume. In small-town Maine, these are things that automatically set you apart.

Over the years, unbeknownst to me at the time, many of my teachers had figured out that something "wasn't right at home." It was a difficult position for them to be in, since they couldn't exactly prove it. I never came to school bruised, I was always clean and well-dressed, and other than stealing food and having occasional dizzy spells, there wasn't a whole lot off about me. I was a very good student, and I had enough friends by the time I got to high school to be considered socially capable (though I had always preferred the company of adults). I was certainly a little odd—what with my *Leave It to Beaver* wardrobe and book reports on *Profiles in Courage*, but I didn't appear to be truly dysfunctional.

Cass, however, was not content to just wonder. And she risked her job to save me.

The fall of my last year of middle school, our class went on some kind of rural expedition that was meant to build character and encourage us to challenge ourselves. A kind of emotional fortification before we were lobbed into high school and peak puberty. It was the first year that Cass had attended this retreat as a chaperone, and she clearly had some apprehensions. With her not-a-strand-out-of-place hair and tailored wardrobe, she was simply too fabulous to be mucking about in the woods with a bunch of off-the-leash preteen girls. Despite my similarly neat-and-tidy wardrobe, I was appreciative of the trip. It meant a few days away from home. That in and of itself made it worth trading my sensible black pumps for sensible black flats.

Though I had no plans to get in a canoe or scale a rock wall, I knew it would be satisfying to observe my peers do so. Many of them had probably never had the kind of adrenaline rush that I lived with every single day, growing up in an unpredictable environment. I never sought thrills, because just surviving was a rush enough for me.

Cass and I, partners in crime as we were, set the tone for the trip as we were packing up the bus. She watched me traipsing across the parking lot with my two suitcases and cackled heartily.

"We're only going to be gone a few days," she said, hoisting them into the back.

I put my hands on my pencil-skirt-clad hips, half-feigning indignation, "Hey! Remember who brought the hairdryer!"

She smiled affectionately at me, then gave me a wink, "I know, *dahhhling*," she trilled, gesturing wildly toward the bus. "Now go on!"

In my middle-school diary, which I dug out for the purpose of telling this story, there's a rather emotional passage where I describe walking back from a campfire alongside Mrs. McCue and blurting out—with the endearing awkwardness of a preteen girl, I imagine—that I wished she was my mother. She put her arm around my shoulder and said that she'd always be there for me, no matter what. Neither of us spoke, and I realized she was trying not to cry.

I HAD ALREADY BEGUN TO feel that my own mother was dead. She was supposedly—as it had been not-so-tenderly put by several relatives—"on her way out." As fate would have it, the very next summer, my mother was still alive, and I found myself once again dwelling in a cabin in the Maine woods. But instead of doing team-building exercises, I was there on a performing arts scholarship.

The summer-long camp was, primarily, for rich "outta state" kids, and the high tuition meant it had never even been on my radar until someone nominated me for a scholarship. The thought of being away from home for an entire summer was breathtaking enough on its own, but to also be studying dance, music, and theater—plus engaging in summer-camp traditions—seemed too good to be true. That summer was the first time in my young life that I felt like I could be myself free from ridicule. I blossomed both in terms of honing my talents and discovering new ones, and becoming socially confident. For the first time in my life, my hard work was praised. I got the lead in the camp production of *Guys and Dolls*. Well, Sky Masterson—one of the male leads (my voice was deeper than most of the boys at camp, who had barely hit puberty). We even cut off a few snips of my hair to glue on some side burns each night during the show's run, which at the time felt very professional to me. The girls I bunked with were all smart, funny, and easily more talented than I was—but we all got along fabulously. My bunkmate, Eve, and I spent many an entertaining evening performing for the others as we imagined conversations between my Eleanor Roosevelt and Virginia Woolf finger-puppets.

That summer also instilled in me the desire to attend Sarah Lawrence. My favorite camp counselor—the young, gifted, gorgeous woman at the center of every summer-camp teen soap ever written, I'm sure—attended the college. Naturally, my preteen mind rationalized that Sarah Lawrence would be the perfect place for me if I wanted to grow up to be just like her.

Growing up seemed a very vague, faraway concept that summer, though. I had confided to the camp's founder that my home situation was as complicated as she had suspected. With each week that passed, that magical summer dwindling right before my eyes, I became more and more anxious. She, unbeknownst to me, had a social work background, and she proved to be a very comforting presence. She was also very supportive when Cass, who had worried about me once school ended and she couldn't keep an eye on me anymore, wanted to visit.

I remember that when she showed up, all my friends thought she was my mom. I didn't correct them. I felt guilty for lying, but for one day I pretended that it was the truth. For one day, I felt like I *had* a mom.

As it happened, while I was lying to my friends in Bunkaroo, my real Mum rallied. By some yet-to-be-explained medical miracle, she didn't die. But she wasn't exactly what you'd call alive, either. She certainly wasn't capable of—or even interested in—being anyone's mother. I had realized by that point that not all of her faltering came from her eating disorder. It went back further than that, to that dynamic she was stuck in with her own mother—with whom I was currently living. In the months after my mother came home and I did not, I grappled with two competing feelings toward her: resentment and empathy. I was angry with her because I felt as though I didn't have a mother. At the same time, as I woke up every morning in the house where she had been thrown against doors, walked by the room where she had desperately hidden vomit in dresser drawers, I realized that when she had been my age she'd felt motherless, too. She probably still did.

Cass began to sense my disquietude and would have just as well tossed me into her gray pickup truck and carted me off to her house in a grand gesture of "I'M YOUR MOM NOW!"—if it wasn't for Nana's rancor toward her. And me. I've found that people are generally willing to admit that parents can abuse children, but they seem to think grandparents are incapable. It's as though they forget that grandparents are parents, and that cycles of abuse don't necessarily end when children grow up. As an adult, I've come to understand that as terrifying as it all felt, the anger was never really about me. And although it felt directed toward me, it wasn't as personal as it felt. Because I wasn't really a person at all.

I was unable to understand the nuances of all this as a young adult. Honestly, I'm not even sure I understand it much better now. Nana's anger preceded me by decades and had little to do with me, even though I got the brunt of it. Of course, it didn't help that she would routinely gaslight me—sometimes even mid-confrontation. Eventually, I wised up and got a tape recorder and recorded her doing it. It wasn't necessarily that I wanted to prove it to anyone else; it was mostly for me. It was my tether to reality, proof that I wasn't making it up or imagining it.

Cass believed me, though, even before I supplied her with hard evidence, because of one instance in particular when I'd hid in my bedroom and called her. The kicker was, Nana was downstairs listening on the other line, gathering intel, I suppose.

"Maybe you should sleep with a knife under your pillow," Cass said, her voice crackling through the phone. Tears squeezed between my face and the receiver as I sat shaking on my bed, letting her voice ground me to a reality I was no longer sure I could survive in.

The next morning, I woke up draped in certitude. I packed a suitcase, slung my backpack over my shoulder, put on my favorite pair of black pumps, and walked to school. When I arrived, suitcase in tow, I stood in the doorway of Cass's classroom. She looked up from her desk and stared at me.

I squared my shoulders and said, simply, "I don't care where I go tonight, but I'm not going back there."

She nodded, then stood without saying a word. She unlocked a small storage closet behind her desk and gestured for me to put my suitcase in it. I did, then headed to class, as though nothing important had happened.

From there, everything unraveled quickly. The life that had wound me up so tightly for almost sixteen years unspooled with the tiniest tug of a loose thread.

A series of screaming matches ensued. I sat on Cass's couch, and she held my hand as I fielded a series of irate telephone calls. Even though I hadn't lived with my mother for several years, she had come to resent the school's meddling, and I suspect it had a lot more to do with her secrets than mine. I don't think she particularly cared where I lived. She just didn't want whatever I did to interfere with her life.

While I saw Cass during those years as a surrogate mother, as an older woman whom I could look up to and confide in, reviewing it now I see that the greatest lesson she taught me was compassion for my own mother. Had my mother been in a situation where people were rooting for her to have more good days than bad ones, to get the help she needed, people who would stand by her even when things got hard, wouldn't her life—wouldn't my life—have been so very different?

In Cass, I had been trying to fill a mother-shaped void inside of me that only seemed to grow larger and more unruly as I aged. I had mistakenly assumed that as I approached adulthood, that void would close up. If anything, it expanded like the cosmos in a shattering smash of a new universe.

Sixteen was the age of my anxiety, but for the first time in my young life, many of the anxieties were totally age-appropriate: SAT prep, prom tears, a rollicking driver's education, boys who climbed out bathroom windows during study hall and girls who wrote mean things about me on the walls of bathroom stalls, late-night confessionals in my best friend's car over an underscore of bands with names like Something Corporate, and trying to learn how to smoke a cigarette on the beach as the salt air competed for space in my lungs. So many things about growing up, about acting my age instead of someone twice as old, were never the sweet performances of youth I'd hoped they'd be. My friends were all breaking free of their parental control, and together we ran with adolescent fearlessness toward the thrilling promise of adulthood. But when they turned around, someone was always there to keep an eye on them. When I turned around, there was nothing but an empty road.

I hadn't run away without a plan, though. For several weeks prior, I'd been taking shelter in my upstairs bedroom with—it's true—a phone book, pulled from beneath the cushions of a kitchen chair, where they had been methodically stacked for years. I flipped through the yellow pages and called every single attorney in the county one after the other.

I've always been a thorough researcher, so it didn't take me long to come across the concept of emancipation. But most of the preliminary Google searches brought back results concerning young actors who wanted to side-step child labor laws or escape their parent-managers, who were cramping their style and stealing their money.

None of that pertained to me; I'd gravitated toward it as a possible solution because I didn't want my younger brother, who still lived with my parents, to have his life upended by whatever action I took. This was a lofty judgment for a fifteen-year-old to consider. In the midst of midterms, one-act play competitions, and SATs. I was trying to grasp legal jargon and figure out how much money I would need to have saved up to support myself until I graduated.

Once word got out that I was essentially a fugitive living in Mrs. McCue's attic, I suppose anyone who had seen me as a bit odd may have felt somewhat gratified. I was the first to admit that the situation was unusual. Though I was incredibly thankful for Cass and her family, I struggled to understand why other adults in my life hadn't stepped in, and why they had been bystanders or enablers for so long. Part of it was down to Cass specifically. Many years after she'd taken me in, she found a section of the Teacher's Handbook that explicitly forbade teachers to "befriend" students in any way, shape, or form. When she told me this, I was dismayed to think that she'd been so close to ruining her career on my account, but she only laughed. As far as she was concerned, it was pretty simple: I needed her help. "Even if I'd known about that rule," she told me, "I would have broken it."

As grateful as I was that Cass didn't have regrets, her revelation gave me some much-needed insight into why other adults affiliated with the schools I'd attended may not have intervened, even if they'd wanted to. Thinking back, I recalled a few vague but comforting memories of a teacher's aide named Meredith. I was eight years old when I knew her, and for awhile I wondered if she hadn't been real at all, if I'd just manufactured her, like an imaginary friend of sorts. So when I was in my early twenties, I decided to use my Internet sleuthing skills to try to find her. Given how much time had elapsed, I was terrified that I would find an obituary, and that in my haste to save my own life I would have missed my chance to thank someone who had made me feel like there was reason to save it.

As it turned out, Meredith lived a little over an hour away from me. Having found an address to which I could send a letter, I wrote to her. I didn't expect that she would remember me, and I certainly didn't expect her to write back inviting me to visit. But she did.

She was exactly as I remembered her, which was so strange, because I was nothing like how she remembered me. And she did remember me. As we ate lunch on their porch, Meredith said that she and her husband had often wondered what had become of me. I gave them the highlights of my heavy story, thankful we were eating light summer salads, and when I reached the end I couldn't help but ask them if they ever suspected what I was dealing with at home.

"You were a shy, unhappy little girl," Meredith said, her eyes glistening with unshed tears. "I just wanted to take you home with me. I remember saying to you, 'If you need to talk, or tell me things, you can.' But I never knew how bad it was."

So, aside from those who knew but could not do anything, I can only assume there were other adults whose experiences echoed Meredith's: they may have suspected, but didn't know the extent of the problems I confronted. I can understand why, too: I may have been shy and unhappy, but I was also a stellar student who didn't cause a lick of trouble. Perhaps I didn't exactly make an effort to seem less odd, but I did make a concerted effort to appear completely in control at all times—which was far more about reassuring myself than about settling anyone else's worries.

This effort was remarkably successful—most of the time. The one incident I remember specifically where the veneer may have been compromised occurred at a choir concert when I was fourteen. Directly beforehand, Nana had ambushed me; blindsided, I had a panic attack backstage and hyperventilated so hard I lost consciousness. Consequently, I was carted off in an ambulance in front of the whole school—but by the following week the teachers had all agreed that it had been "an asthma attack." In the ambulance, Nana had insisted on riding shotgun so she could interrogate the paramedics for the entire twenty-minute ride to the hospital, throwing in the occasional jab at semiconscious me. When I came to, the paramedic asked me, in a low, level voice, if Nana was hurting me. I couldn't speak through the oxygen mask, so I locked pleading, tearful eyes with him and nodded my head wildly. He nodded solemnly and shot a glance toward the front seat, as if he were expecting her head to twist around like the girl's in that scene of *The Exorcist*.

I don't know what, if anything, of our turbulent ride was relayed to the ER physician—but the note in my medical record represents another occasion upon which the health-care system inevitably failed me:

Date: 12/06/2005
Blood Pressure: 140/86
Heart Rate: 115 bpm

HISTORY OF PRESENT ILLNESS:
Chief complaint: ANXIETY AND DIFFICULTY BREATHING.

This started today (couldn't breathe while performing with the choir). Is still present but is improving. Has been upset. Has had suicidal thoughts (in the remote past). Has briefly considered suicide. The patient has had anxiety. She has experienced situational problems related to school (family).

In spite of these notes, I was discharged home—to my parents, with whom I had not lived for two years. Shortly thereafter, I was returned to Nana's house. The incident was never discussed, and there was no follow-up. About a month later I tried to hang myself with a dog leash. Nana was on the phone in the other room, yelling at my mother—probably about something that had happened twenty years ago. I put the radio on and fumbled my way through getting the leash over my head, tears streaming down my face as I stared somewhat vacantly at the wall. Despite the tears, I was calm and methodical about it, because it felt like the right thing to do.

I closed my eyes and stepped off the top step—then nothing. Failure. I was still there. I hadn't planned well enough, and my body dropped to the floor in a heap. I didn't get up right away, but just stayed there staring at the pockmarked ceiling. My grandmother yelled to me from the next room, "Stop making all that goddamn noise!"

Years later, when doctors and others would try to blame my myriad constitutional symptoms on my childhood, I'd want to scream at them that they should have believed me when I said I needed help. That they should have believed my mother and my grandmother when *they* had needed help. But they didn't. If they wanted to imply that I had in some way succumbed to the poison of those early experiences, I'd have to beg to differ: when I realized they wouldn't, or couldn't, help me, I started trying to find a way to save myself.

Before I could do that, though, I had to figure out how to protect someone other than myself: my little brother. I'd been living with Nana for a couple of years by then, and it was really that environment that I was trying to escape. Though going back to my parents wasn't a healthy choice for me, my brother was getting his needs met there. Even at fifteen, I understood that the foster care system would have eaten us both alive. We would have no doubt been packed in with hundreds of other kids, waiting to be adopted, and the fact that he had autism practically guaranteed that he'd be waiting indefinitely. The truth, though it might have been hard for me to understand, was that he loved my parents and they loved him. I was the irreconcilable difference.

But emancipation would leave my brother untouched, and it allowed me the legal freedom necessary to make decisions that were in favor of getting help (such as seeing a therapist, which my family had refused to allow me to do, for fear of secrets being let out).

The lawyers I called agreed with me, as it turned out: the only problem was that it was election year, and they were all running for district attorney. That meant they weren't going to be taking on any new cases. They all gave me someone else's phone number and their best wishes. I kept calling. All I needed was one yes.

And Mr. Fenig gave it to me.

I'D NEVER REALLY KNOWN ANY lawyers before I met Mr. Fenig. When we first spoke on the phone, he seemed intrigued—and, he wasn't running for DA.

One spring day after school, Cass and her husband took me to his office, which was conveniently located near the district court. He was going to talk to all of us, but separately. His office was exactly what I had envisioned an attorney's office would be: shiny mahogany and enough burgundy to make you regret whatever it is you did to wind up there. I didn't realize how tall he was until he rose from behind his equally formidable desk, which was, I'm sure, crafted from a grade of wood commensurate to his profession. He was a distinguished man of late middle age who spoke with a clipped baritone, which seemed like it belonged to the canon of every courtroom drama I'd seen. A veteran of the law though he was, he still seemed a bit perplexed by my presence—a fact I gleaned from the way he would narrow his eyes at me with a half-smile that seemed to imply amusement.

He explained that getting emancipated would be more paperwork than anything else. When I turned sixteen, I would file a petition with the probate court. Included with this would be a statement, to be read by a judge, that would explain why I was seeking emancipation and

outline my plan for living if my request was granted. I presumed that
he explained the same to Cass and her husband when it was their
scene in the *Law and Order* episode my life had become.

Over the next couple of weeks, I wrote what was arguably going
to be the most important essay of my school career, for which I would
receive no grade. I brought that, as well as my petition, to the probate
court on my sixteenth birthday.

Soon after I submitted my paperwork, I was called in to Mr.
Fenig's office, where he accused me of not understanding the proper
procedure—of not appreciating the law: it had been made perfectly
clear that I had to write the statement by myself. So why, he wondered, had I clearly had an adult write it for me?

I hadn't had an adult so much as spell-check the damned thing.
I'd written every word myself. He shook his head, dropping the
statement onto a pile of papers on his desk. "No judge will believe a
sixteen-year-old kid wrote that," he said. When the school supplied
writing samples as proof, he conceded that perhaps it was possible I
had written the statement after all. Still, it probably wouldn't hurt to
make it a little less eloquent.

Within just a few weeks, my parents were served with papers and
a court date was set: June 19, 2007.

This date landed right in the middle of finals. To be perfectly
honest, I hadn't expected to get a date so quickly. Midsummer seemed
hopeful. For several reasons, logistical and personal, I had hoped it
would be after school let out, because I didn't want anyone to know
about it. My close friends knew, of course, and were supportive of
me, but I didn't need the entire town to be in on it.

Unfortunately, there are no secrets in tight-knit communities.
Even before the day came, I found myself at the mercy of small-town
gossip. Despite the fact that I had been elected class president, was
on the National Honor Society, and ranked fifth in my class, people
suddenly didn't want their kids associating with me because I was
"divorcing my parents." School administrators, who had no idea what
to do with me, started to treat me like a delinquent, when I didn't
have so much as a detention on my record.

Luckily, the teachers were, for the most part, very accommodat-
ing. They allowed me to take a few of my finals early so that I could

leave before the afternoon session on the day of my hearing. Still, I failed my math final: it's the only test I've ever failed in my academic career.

As pursuant to the court, someone from the school had to accompany me. That's how Kim, the first-name-basis guidance counselor who ultimately led me to Jane, got involved.

My hearing was supposed to be in the early afternoon, but when we arrived at the courthouse, we were informed that a particularly nasty divorce hearing had gone into overtime; as a result, my case was pushed back on the docket by a few hours. That was all fine by me, as I'd been hoping to have time to prepare myself, though I didn't know exactly what I was preparing for.

I'd been told it would go like this: my parents would show up, and we'd yell and scream for a few hours—which was pretty normal, only this time we'd have an audience. Mr. Fenig sat me in a tiny room with a tall, thin window overlooking the street in front of the courthouse. I looked through the venetian blinds, waiting to see my parents walk up the steps. Kim brought me a glass of water. I shuffled the papers that contained my written statement. I asked Mr. Fenig if there was anything I should know going in. He stood in the entryway with his hands stuffed into the pockets of his suit jacket. "Answer the judge's questions, read your statement—and don't cry," he said, checking his watch.

When my case finally came up, there was a moment of panicked silence as we realized that my parents had not yet arrived. An eerie sense of relief mixed with disappointment came over me. When I look back on it now, I realize that at some level I had wanted that confrontation with them—I wanted the resulting closure. I was making a very definitive decision about my life, and even if that decision was to ceremoniously cut them out of it, they were still my parents. I still wanted them to care.

Out of the corner of my eye, I saw my parents' car pull up in front of the courthouse. My father threw it into park and didn't even shut off the ignition. He emerged from the idling car, walked up the front steps, then returned moments later, speeding off down the street.

Confused, I turned to look up at Mr. Fenig in the doorway, but he wasn't there. When he reappeared a few minutes later, he held a piece of paper in his hand, which he dropped on the table in front of me the way you might a napkin.

"They aren't going to contest it," he said simply, "All you have to do now is go in there, read your statement, and keep from crying. You'll be granted emancipation by default."

I nodded, stilling myself. He was right. If I wanted a judge to see me as being grown up enough to take care of myself, I had to keep it together. Life was no doubt going to be full of unexpected twists. I had to prove that I was stable enough to handle them, change course, and keep going. I had done my research. I'd come prepared. I believed, as did Cass, as did my lawyer, that I was making the most reasonable choice for myself that I could in a situation where, really, there was never going to be a good choice. No choice would have been easy, but I had plenty of evidence to support the high probability of a negative outcome if I made the choice to stay.

I made the short walk down the hallway from the waiting room to the courtroom in my ill-fitting, secondhand suit, the pencil skirt wrinkled even though I'd tried to smooth it out with the spine of my biology textbook in the girls' bathroom before I'd left school that morning. I knew I didn't have a lot of data on the outcome for emancipated minors. There were more unknown variables than known variables. I just had to hope that whenever I solved the equation, at some later point in my life, the answer would be positive. Or maybe I'd never get an answer, but be doomed to be the asymptote, always approaching—but never quite reaching—infinity.

The rest of my life, whatever it was to become, was decided in less than twenty minutes. I'd been gearing up for weeks, trying to mentally prepare myself for what I had only assumed would be the most profoundly soul-shattering confrontation of my life—and then, nothing. I'd waited longer for a pizza than I had for my freedom. It was the calmest, most reasonable, well-paced event of my entire life thus far. Just as Mr. Fenig had instructed, I went into the courtroom, took the oath on a tattered county courthouse Bible, and numbly read my statement.

I had read my statement, rehashed versions of it, so many times in the previous few weeks that it had ceased to feel like it belonged to me. When I finished, the judge complimented my writing. I was immediately thrown off by this; it wasn't like I was in an oration competition. I sheepishly thanked her. She questioned me about my plans, and I explained, in a measured, slightly deferential tone, that I was going to live with Cass and her family, stay in school, and keep working my strange little part-time jobs (which would be full time on weekends, holidays, and summer vacation). I would use my eligibility for Medicaid insurance coverage to, first and foremost, get a therapist, so I could become as well-adjusted as possible before college—which, I added, I was already preparing for by taking college-level classes; I had a stack of scholarship applications already piling up. After a beat she nodded, seemingly satisfied, and wished me luck. I was startled when she banged her gavel, which I hadn't actually expected her to do.

Out on the sidewalk, Mr. Fenig shook my hand and congratulated me, though it seemed a strange thing to be congratulated on. He gave me his best wishes and, with a confident stride, headed back to his office. I'm pretty sure there had been *Judge Judy* episodes that had gone on longer than my hearing.

"Do you want to get ice cream?" Kim, the guidance counselor, piped as we sat in uncomfortable silence in her car. I must have looked at her with abject horror, because she returned an apologetic glance and started the car.

She pulled out of the parking lot and headed back to town as I rolled the car window down, gulping down a lungful of fresh air. I knew this was the last moment I would have to breathe easy for many years to come. After a few minutes of uneasy silence, Kim asked me where I wanted to go.

I choked up and said, though I had no idea what it meant anymore, "*Home.*"

YEARS LATER, WHEN I FOUND myself back in Maine, terrified and sick, the only thing I could think to do was call Jane. When I walked in to her office again, she looked a bit sad, wearing an expression of mild disappointment. It was like the face you might make upon realizing you'd stumbled across your favorite movie on television—forty-five minutes in.

I had returned to her office pallid, thin, soft-spoken, and tearful—merely a husk of the girl she'd sat across from three years before when I'd first walked into her office. I would like to say simply that we resumed our sessions, but the truth is, I think we started all over again. I wondered if her faint look of disappointment wasn't directed at me. She couldn't hide her shock when I walked into her office again: I had shed so much weight that my hip bones jutted out, two angular shivs, above the waistband of my jeans. Her face had contorted into a brief grimace that she was quick to cover up, but I'd seen it. I'd felt it.

I lay curled up on the couch in her office during our sessions purely out of exhaustion. I simply could not sit upright for fifty minutes straight. She would sit in her chair by the window with her thermos of what I always assumed was herbal tea, and calmly listen while I wept. For several months that winter I saw her fairly regularly—once, maybe twice, during the week. Sometimes she was the only person I spoke to for weeks on end.

CHAPTER 4

If you desire healing,
let yourself fall ill.

—Rumi

HARRY HARLOW, A BEHAVIORIST WORKING in a lab in the 1950s, wanted to better understand the bond between babies and their primary caregivers, i.e., their mothers. He couldn't use actual human infants, because he knew that if he deprived them of their mothers as much as he needed to for his study, they'd die—an outcome that would do absolutely nothing to advance his research career. So instead, he used rhesus monkeys.

Essentially, what Harlow did was construct a physical situation for the monkeys that would represent what would happen to human babies who weren't held or cuddled. Perhaps these babies were in orphanages or were otherwise being institutionally cared for, and were therefore neglected. It was also possible that they had just been born to parents who, for myriad reasons, could not or would not hold them beyond what was absolutely necessary for transportation. Harlow built apparatuses out of wire. Some of the apparatuses had a little plush fur around them that made them kind of cozy, like a mother monkey presumably would be. Others had nothing: just cold, hard wires. Both kinds were terrifying to look at, but the metal ones were particularly unsettling. Those, of course, were the

ones that Harlow fed the monkeys from, through a bottle affixed to
the wires.

And wouldn't you know it, these poor baby monkeys, who had
been taken from their mothers not even a day after birth, only used
the wire mother for sustenance. The rest of the time, they huddled
pathetically against the warm, "cozy" one, trying not to lose their
minds. Sadly, most of them did lose their minds. They were being
fed, and therefore weren't in danger of starving to death, but they
were being starved in another way. The monkeys were driven into a
spiral of anxiety and depression so severe that they could never survive outside of the fucked-up little experiment Harlow had created.
They had been profoundly damaged by the separation and the conse-
quent hell in which they had been raised.

These monkeys, Harlow wrote, "became bizarre later in life.
They engaged in stereotyped behavior patterns, such as clutching
themselves and rocking constantly back and forth, and exhibited excessive and misdirected aggression."

You might be surprised to learn that many of these monkeys, despite their maladjustment, did actually grow up to be adult monkeys,
though. As adult monkeys, they mated though often with signifi
cant difficulty. Harlow wrote that many of the monkeys had no idea
how to copulate, describing one female as presenting for sex with "a
posture in which only her heart was in the right place."

Despite their initial confusion, these females could, and did, bear
offspring. And although they may have survived their unloving environment in the sterile safety of a laboratory, their young were not so
fortunate. The "motherless mothers," as Harlow put it, "proved to be
very inadequate."

The monkeys he had raised in isolation "tended to be either indifferent or abusive toward their babies" as mothers. "The indifferent mothers," Harlow wrote, "did not nurse, comfort, or protect their
young, but they did not harm them"—at least not intentionally. Some
of the monkey moms, however, were more aggressive. Harlow even
went so far as to call them abusive. These monkey mothers were
known to bite their infants, "to the point that many of them died."

The ethics of Harlow's experiment have been constantly debated
since it was completed. It's easy to understand why it messed with

people so much to see those hopeless little monkeys. Baby primates, after all, are just human-looking enough, with their big eyes, that we anthropomorphize them and empathize with them. We feel for them, not unlike the way we would feel if we were seeing a human baby, and the experiment itself somehow feels inhumane.

I was first exposed to Harlow's work in earnest in a psychology lecture at Sarah Lawrence my freshman year, with the dulcet tones of that lovely Scottish prof Elizabeth Johnston leading us down to the depths of depravity. I remember reading *Love at Goon Park* as assigned reading that semester and often finding myself in tears. I felt bad for the little monkeys, I told myself. They were so cute, and vulnerable, and doomed. Harlow had done this terrible, terrible thing to them. In the name of science, yes—I did understand that much. But still, they were just little babies. And they were scared and alone and clearly in so much pain. An inextricable pain. Maybe not quite a physical pain, but I could see it in their eyes as they looked out wildly from their cages.

The day in class when we watched Harlow's films of the monkeys, we were all eerily silent, transfixed by the horror. Abruptly cut, grainy, black-and-white shots of the monkeys injuring themselves in the name of self-soothing, desperately suckling from the wire-mother, always trying to keep even just a little toe on the warm, cozy mother beside it. Their big, dark eyes stared up at me from where they clung to that pathetic piece of fabric that even they must have known wasn't really mommy. It wasn't really anything—but it had to be enough.

Much to my chagrin, I began to cry. After a few minutes, I casually walked out of the classroom and down the hall to the small bathroom around the corner. I locked myself in and sank to the floor, biting my hand to keep from making any noise.

I looked up at nothing, eyes wide, swallowing those big, rolling sobs as my heart shuttered closed in fearful recognition. In the beginning, it had been the sight of Harlow's monkeys suffering that had brought me to tears. But in that moment, the anguish I felt was my own.

THE SUMMER BEFORE MY SENIOR year of high school was a strange one. Freshly liberated, and determined to make as much money as possible so that I could unequivocally attend whichever college I was accepted to, I took on a series of odd jobs. Odd in the sense that they were a mishmash of temporary employment, and also odd in the sense that they were really unusual. The first involved living and working at one of the many Victorian inns in town, the second, starring in a summer stock theater production.

The arrangement was fine until midway through the summer, when the innkeeper's son fell ill. The innkeeper announced that she needed to travel to be with him, then left me to run the place alone for a few weeks. I balked at first—I was in high school, after all—but she was either confident in me or desperate enough to be with her son that she left anyway. My money has always been on the latter.

I was also still attempting to get through rehearsals of the show I'd been cast in, which had an outdoor performance schedule coming up that was more rigorous than I had anticipated. I'd just thought it would be a fun way to make some money, but having one of the lead roles meant that my life that summer boiled down to rehearsing and turning over beds at the inn nonstop. I'd sing scales as I trudged up and down the back staircase from the bedrooms to the laundry, and it probably warded off as many potential guests as it did ghosts (the place *was* haunted—but then again, what old house in New England isn't?).

Once the innkeeper had left and it was truly down to me, I began a manic-frenzy of playing dual roles: by day, *Abby, a twenty-three-year-old linguistics major at Middlebury*! to the guests at the inn, and sweet ingenue at night once the show opened. Somehow, I pulled it off—but not without the price of pure emotional and physical exhaustion.

On top of everything else that had befallen me that summer, I'd started to have trouble keeping my sheets clean. My periods had always been heavy—no matter where I'd been sleeping over the years, I'd carried with me the fear of bleeding on someone's linens. But they now seemed to be getting mercilessly painful. I quite reasonably chalked it up to stress. In any case, as soon as the innkeeper returned, I left in a rather ungraceful haste, slinking off into the summer heat with my soiled sheets like an estrogen-rich Quasimodo.

When I took the job at the inn, I'd been living with Cass's family for a little over a year. Although she'd expected that I'd continue living there until I graduated, her daughter—who had, almost overnight, become a teenager—had started to need Cass in the push-pull way that all teenage girls do, and I felt very much an intruder in that sacred space. When my job at the inn, and the summer, drew to an end, I spent a few weeks living out of my car (a Ford I affectionately called Harrison) that I'd come by thanks to an elderly gentleman named Walter.

Although Walter had been in my life since the day I was born, I did not really get to know him well until I was a teenager on the lam. Walter had been in a long-term relationship with my grandmother since before I came along, and he was always sort of on the periphery of my life. To many who knew him, he was an imposing figure: tall, serious, bespectacled. He had come of age the same way many men of his generation did: in Germany during World War II, when he was practically still a teenager. And like many men of his era, he didn't talk about it much.

When he came home from the front, Walter traded the chaotic death of wartime for the more sterile, controlled kind of demise to be found in the city morgue: he became an undertaker. It was only after years of trying to patch bodies back together that he decided to go into law enforcement, hoping that he might save some people from the kind of exsanguinatory fate he knew awaited them on the slab.

When I was a kid, I was expressly told that Walter didn't like children, which was why he didn't have any. I didn't find that too hard to believe: although I was never frightened of Walter when I came in from playing to find him seated at my grandmother's kitchen table, I was a little wary of him. Even still, his tight-lipped reticence fascinated me. He didn't say much, but he was a constant, quiet presence. He and my grandmother never lived together—he came and went as he pleased—but he was always around to mow her lawn or shovel us out after a blizzard. His frequent presence was a given, even if I didn't know if that meant he was there for me.

It was Walter who found, and bought, Harrison for me. This was on two conditions: first, that the car remain in his name until I could afford to pay for the insurance myself, at which time he'd sell it to me, and second, that he was going to teach me to drive. The prospect of being taught to drive by an ex-cop was a little terrifying, but I wasn't about to look a gift horse in the mouth. So when Harrison came into my life, he brought Walter—the real Walter that I had not known—with him.

After school, Walter would pick me up and fold himself into the front seat of the Taurus. He'd firmly instruct me as we drove through town, but he never raised his voice or demeaned me in any way if I made a mistake. He would *suggest* that I stop speeding, and made a point to inform me that I was not, under any circumstances, to open the car's sunroof. When I asked why, he answered by telling me about a time during his years on the force when he'd spent several hours by the side of the highway looking for heads when a convertible full of teenagers had been in an accident.

"They had, of course, been decapitated," he'd said, glancing at me sideways from the passenger seat, and then slowly looking up at the sunroof.

"So, I don't want to see that open . . ." he'd said, clearing his throat, "or heads—as they say—will roll."

I turned to look at him, still trying to keep one eye on the road. He was grinning in his dark way, but gestured for me to pay attention to driving. Our shared macabre sense of humor got us through the agony of my driver's education, and by the end of it, not only did I have my driver's license and a safe vehicle—but I had a semblance of a grizzled grandpa. If Harrison wouldn't start, or it overheated on a backroad, I could call him, and he'd lumber over to fix it, sending me on my way after leaving a $20 bill in the cupholder.

While Walter and I talked plenty about mortuary science (he would have liked to see me go into it, I know), we hardly ever spoke about anything else that happened in either of our lives. But one day I asked him why he got me the car. It wasn't that I was ungrateful. Quite the contrary: I was just surprised.

"I knew if I didn't, no one else would," he said simply, the words blunt but softened by the warble of his voice. "You're a good kid," he added—and that was my answer.

Walter was already an old man when I was born, so by the time I entered adulthood and fell ill, he, too, had entered a more feeble state of existence. Although I had learned, through his patient teaching, how to change a tire on my own, and check the car's fluids, I had a feeling of security knowing that Walter would always pick up the phone. Each year on my birthday, no matter where I was living (and I was almost always living somewhere new), as if by magic I'd get a card from him. Some years his was the only card that came.

The year I turned twenty-five, I did not get a card from him. I had visited him at his home—for the first time in years—a few months before, and he had not been well. Of course, neither was I, but I didn't want him to know that. I spent several hours with him in his old farmhouse, and he spoke more in those hours than he had in the twenty-five years I'd known him. He showed me a picture of his wife, who had died too young of cancer, and whom he had never stopped loving. He showed me the military medals he'd been awarded, photographs of him as a young man in all black, the crisp uniform of an undertaker.

He also told me that it had meant a lot to him to be part of my life when I was a child. I was touched, but also found it curious. I'd been told repeatedly that he didn't like children, had never wanted any, and that the fact that he tolerated me was just the exception to the rule. He got a bit misty-eyed as he explained that was not true in the least: he had been rendered infertile during the war. That was why he had no children.

When he died the following winter, I was quite grief stricken. Walter had not, at any point in my life, been someone I spoke to daily, and aside from that one afternoon where he had told me so much, I still knew very little about him in the grand scheme of things. I'd been grateful to him, and for him, my entire life. And I had a pristine driving record that I chalked up entirely to his teachings. But I had known, on some level, when the birthday card had not come that year, that it meant he would probably die soon. I also knew, from all our conversations about death over the years, in the most scientific of senses, that he had not feared it. He had not wanted me to fear death, either, which was why he spoke about it the way he did.

I realized in the days following Walter's death that he had succeeded in that: it was not my own death that I had feared, but his. When he was truly gone, and I knew that if I called the telephone in that old farmhouse that it would ring and ring into eternity, never reaching him, I came to see that the most valuable thing he gave me was not his help, or his money, or even his kindness, but that he had taught me to take care of myself.

I also inherited an antique embalming kit from him. I can tell you that, circa 1952, the lip color *du jour* for the on-trend corpse was Avon's "Misty Carnation." There were also several typewritten drafts of papers that he had written as head of the mortuary, instructing his charges how to properly handle dead bodies so as not to expose the living to any "pestilences" of "time immemorial." He advises them that they need not fear, because they have the technology and know-how—what he calls "mercifully true science"—to prevent such scourges, so long as they pay attention and heed the facts.

As I drove home with this rather large embalming case (embossed with a gold plate bearing his name) in the front seat, my car bleated incessantly in a misguided attempt to alert me that the "passenger" wasn't belted. I had a good cry thinking about all those times I'd be behind the wheel with Walter in Harrison's passenger seat.

One night, during that summer when Harrison had become a temporary domicile, I was sprawled out in the front seat, staring up into the night sky through the opening in the roof. My dwelling was almost comedically filled with clothes and books, all my worldly belongings—and then some. I stuck my feet on the dashboard and read under the halo of a streetlamp, trying to find answers in the pages of worn books. I wasn't at ease, but I wasn't exactly afraid, either. I had what I hoped wouldn't turn out to be a Blanche Duboisian reliance on the kindness of strangers, along with reliance on my own strange self to figure out what was next. And for once in my life, I wasn't worried about bleeding all over anyone's Egyptian cotton sheets.

During the run of the show that summer before senior year, I had taken a shine to a woman who worked at the theater named Estelle. She had this air of glamour that made her look wildly out of place in Midcoast Maine, which was probably because she *was* a little out of place there. Like many interesting people, she had once lived in New York City—a fact that dazzled me as much as she'd hoped it would. One night, during the final run of the show, Estelle was taking bobby pins out of my hair after the performance and casually asked me about where I was off to. Overtired but still high-strung, and therefore chatty from the adrenaline, I spat out the not-too-glamorous truth. I've always been a shitty liar when in need of a nap.

Aghast—something that Estelle loved to be, for the sake of tragedy—she blurted out that she had a spare room, the implication being that I should stay with her.

AT THIS POINT, I WAS essentially acting as my own case worker and vetting a potential foster mother. But what do you suppose happens when a pedantic teenage girl, desperate for a family but with no real sense of what family means, sets out to try to forge healthy relationships with adults in her life who should, in theory, care for and about her?

During my unfinished research on maternal attachment at Sarah Lawrence, I read a book postulating that some children who are orphaned or put into foster care seem to possess a peculiar, almost bewitching kind of resilience. Adults are drawn to them in orphanages, in hospitals, in schools, and in care centers. This is how these children survive and sometimes even thrive. They have a certain quality about them that is just a little bit magical.

This reminded me of when I was small, reading well above my grade level, and the school librarian gave me a copy of *Matilda* by Roald Dahl. As most little children are, I was enchanted by the story, but it wasn't until many years later (and years of comparisons being made) that I thought perhaps the librarian had hoped I would identify with Dahl's bookworm. That maybe I would find some hope in it. It's true, Matilda does get her happy ending. Her teacher, Miss Honey, adopts her and it's all quite lovely. Of course, it's all also very convenient, because Miss Honey does not have any children of her own, and Matilda still has plenty of time developmentally to form a strong attachment to her new caregiver.

With a somewhat clumsy flourish, I took Estelle up on her offer and lived there my senior year of high school. Most, if not all, of my memories of her from that time involve standing out on her back porch at dusk watching her smoke a cigarette. I have never in my life met someone who looked as good smoking a cigarette as Estelle did. As detrimental to one's health (and wallet) as smoking may be, Estelle looked like an old Hollywood movie star whenever she held a cigarette between her slim, elegant fingers. Her high, severe cheekbones shaping her face as she inhaled, the glittering assortment of precious stones in her rings catching the rays of fading sun. No doubt she, too, had caught light that way once.

"Don't you just love the pink light, princess?" she'd ask me in her fervent way, her deep, throaty voice cutting through a plume of smoke as she gestured to the haze of light that fell over her yard when the sun went down.

Estelle brought an unchecked intensity to everything in her life that fascinated me, and she could be wonderfully affectionate and supportive. At times, she was a maternal force in my life, something I had desperately needed. When I confessed to her that I was embarrassed by my apparent inability to wear tampons, she sat outside the bathroom door patiently trying to talk me through it.

From day one, Estelle had also taken it upon herself to try to teach me how to be less of a frump. For a young woman who had spent the better part of her childhood undernourished, the weight of puberty was welcomed. I didn't see myself as being especially overweight, but my run-ins with the town gossips at the grocery store kept me abreast of my mother's and grandmother's opinions on the subject, which were pretty fatalistic.

I carried their perception of fault with me, but I suppose I didn't find it enough of a slight to take any action. Still, I was dressing my newly curvaceous body in a never-ending cascade of vintage attire that worked well in theory, but perhaps not for the decade I was actually living in. I didn't care. I loved clothes, and I dressed for myself. Estelle did suggest that perhaps I could try a little harder in terms of pride in presentation, though—especially where my eyebrows were concerned. I can still see her face, her own brows knitted together in concentration—so much so that I was getting a headache just looking at her—as she studied them, a pair of tweezers poised above my face. Ever since the day she plucked them, I've continued to diligently have them waxed and shaped. I've never tried to make them into something that they aren't naturally inclined to be, but Estelle did show me the power of tidying them up a bit.

It might seem like Estelle offered me little of emotional substance, since her focus always seemed to be on appearance. But with my mother and grandmother, that focus had always been laser-sharp, hypercritical, and honestly, very warped. Estelle really was only trying to help, and trying to find a way to forge a bond. We weren't mother and daughter by any stretch—although, whenever she'd be in the position of having to explain who I was or why I was living in her house, she'd sort of wave her pretty hands in my general direction and go, "I'm like, her *mom-thing*."

Mom or not, she tried to impart her decades of feminine wisdom however she could think to do so. Getting dolled up made her feel good, so I think she hoped it might make me feel better, too. As much as I would feel a bit embarrassed if she tried to style my hair or show me a better way to apply makeup, I appreciate now that she was trying to teach me something about living in the world with the body I had. Estelle had an eye for beauty, something I'd learned about her right away when I'd watch her studying the sun as it slinked down over the horizon. But a lot of people can appreciate beauty when it's obvious. Estelle could see something beautiful even when it was obscured, or had been browbeaten into hiding. She could coax beauty out and find a place for it to live, welcomed in the world's empty spaces. Estelle could see the possibility of beauty everywhere. Even in me.

There were certain things about me that she could never understand, or that made her visibly uncomfortable. It seems strange that I could have been intimidating to her emotionally—since she was easily the most ebullient person I've ever known. That was the hardest part of living in so many different houses as a teenager: when someone opens their home to you, they need to know who you are. They want to understand you—if for no other reason than that they can rest assured you aren't going to commit arson or steal their fine china. But there's also an intimate, emotional component to cohabitation, even if you barely talk to each other. I was almost eighteen. My personality changed with the tides, wavering between child and adult. I spent a lot of time emulating women I admired, trying on bits and pieces, running their intonations across my lips like Dusty Rose, trying to find a shade that suited me. And if Estelle had an abundance of anything, it was feelings and lipstick.

Aside from potential splendor, the other thing Estelle was skilled at dragooning from people was emotion. Her rapt attention encouraged more than a few woebegone soliloquies to emerge from me—an adjective she probably planted in my mind. I'd try to make it home from my weekend job on Saturday afternoons so we could listen to Garrison Keillor on *A Prairie Home Companion* together. Well, not together exactly, but in companionable orbit. I was usually in the living room with the radio, reading or working on homework. And she'd be bustling around doing laundry and cooking—almost always cooking. In fact, she had speakers or a radio in just about every room of her house. No matter what room you were in—and even if you were on the porch or in the backyard—on Saturday afternoons you'd hear the tales from Lake Wobegon.

Over the years, I've found that I can't listen to it in her absence. It seems incomplete without her rasping laughter punctuating the broadcast, rising up over the banjo-slaps like steam from the pot of water she'd be toiling over in those warm, drowsy afternoons.

One day, I came home from school to find that Estelle had left my mail on the stairs, the same as she always had. Not that I got a lot of mail, and most of the mail I did receive looked like it had gone through the wringer a few times: returned postage, scribbled out addresses, a lot of question marks next to my name. But on that middling winter-spring day, a large, green envelope with Sarah Lawrence College's logo embossed on it awaited me.

My heart nearly beat out of my chest and I tripped my way up the stairs as I tore into it. I probably used my teeth, my hunger to know its contents tapping into my most primeval needs. I had already been accepted into the other schools I'd applied to: Bryn Mawr, Wells, and the University of Maine, which was my "safety school." Much to my dismay, I'd been waitlisted at Vassar, because they had requested some kind of essay about me be submitted by my mother, which I, for obvious reasons, could not supply. Sarah Lawrence, though, had always been my first choice, ever since that metamorphic summer at camp when I'd taken dance classes from a raven-haired alumna.

Although I'd really had my heart set on the place, I'd had no idea whether I could actually get in. I had, like many other college-hopeful students, taken the SATs not once, but twice, sending my best scores to my chosen institutions of higher learning. I'd received a perfect score on the essay portion of the SATs, which gave me a thrill that was immediately tempered by how poorly I'd performed in the math section. As it turned out, Sarah Lawrence didn't even require you to submit your test scores. And aside from that, it had a self-proclaimed writing-dominant program that weighted one's personal essay heavily. Having written a solid enough essay to convey my readiness at sixteen to care for myself to a judge, I thought it reasonable to hope I could write one to convince an admissions committee of my college readiness. Which, I guess, I did.

Although I had my emancipation document, heavy with its official signage and stamp, tucked away in a box where I didn't look at it unless I had to, my acceptance letter to Sarah Lawrence became my most prized testimony. I flew down the stairs, nearly knocking Estelle over as I skidded into the kitchen, brandishing it proudly. She'd suspected that it was an acceptance letter, but actually seeing it was positively merrymaking.

The next day, I walked into school beaming. I couldn't wait for the principal to make the announcement over the intercom (as he did for every senior once they'd chosen a school, military branch, or other post-high-school vocation). No other students had arrived yet, so I sauntered into my favorite English teacher's classroom. The first bell had yet to ring, and he was alone, sitting at his desk grading papers. I dropped the acceptance letter onto his desk, expecting him to be elated. He looked shocked, lowering his glasses onto the bridge of his nose.

"You got in—?" he asked incredulously. His gaze fell from mine, dropping to the letter as he inspected it more closely. "Oh my God," came his wonder across a single breath. He looked up at me again, a smile breaching his lips, his eyes sparkling over his spectacles. "You did it. You got in. You actually got in."

I blinked, a bit startled by his doubt. But as I watched him processing the news, I realized that his scruples were not unlike those of any other grown-up who had hesitated to believe me, or in me. I didn't want to think my faith in him had been misplaced. He had been the one who had taught us all about Joseph Campbell's archetype of the Hero's Journey—leaving the known world for the unknown, enduring the struggle, becoming transformed—and, in the end, attaining the much-sought-after reward. It was the most ubiquitous story in human history, and he'd been the one who had taught it to us. So how could he not see what seemed so obvious to me? That letter was my ultimate boon. Whether or not he, or anyone else, had even been aware of the strange little saga I'd been living, he couldn't deny the triumph in its conclusion.

After all, he was holding the proof in his hands.

CHAPTER 5

The body never lies.

—Martha Graham, *Blood Memory*

THE DISCOURSE ON THE ILLS of women, not just in the psychological and medical community, but culturally, almost always includes a diagnosis of hysteria. Even before it had a name, the concept of what hysteria would become was integral to how women were perceived: they were emotionally labile to a pathological degree, or vulnerable to demonic possession or other manipulations by unseen evils, or perceived as being more likely to sin (intentionally, through their wicked witchery, or unintentionally, because of their fragility or stupidity relative to men).

In the annals of not-that-distant psychology, Sigmund Freud—a nonfriend to women if there ever was one—published a case study about a woman he called Dora that would become one of the most influential case studies ever to grace our contemporary understanding of hysteria. Dora had come of age in the mid-1890s—a period in history when women were constrained physically not just by the limits imposed on them by the men in their lives, but also through the en vogue fashions of the day, which relied heavily on corsets. Whether women were seeking permission or approval, their fathers or uncles or brothers, and eventually their husbands, had a great deal of power over them. For those who began to exhibit functional neurological or

other symptoms, physicians and psychiatrists—who were also predominantly male—were thrown into the mix, too.

Among those men who sought to understand hysteria—which
they believed to be strictly a female disease—Freud's theory seemed
to be the one that stuck, and it has remained part of the public consciousness ever since. Eighteen case studies—a small sample size,
really—were the basis for his belief that the sole cause of hysteria
was a sexual trauma that took place during a woman's childhood. But
a woman only became hysterical if she repressed those memories, so
that they were left to fester in her unconscious mind. Her first major
hysterical "episode" was usually "triggered" by a sexual experience
that she had at or after puberty, and Freud believed that the severity
of symptoms was directly linked to the frequency with which she'd
been sexually abused. He eventually revised his theory to add that
an actual sexual experience during childhood wasn't even a prereq-
uisite for hysteria: if a woman had so much as imagined that she'd
had one—or, perhaps, had the memory planted—that was enough
to cause hysteria. His theory for curing hysteria, then, was to use the
principles of psychoanalysis to help the woman recover the traumatic
memories she'd repressed—whether they were based on real events
or her "fantasies"—and acknowledge them, at which point her physical symptoms would be resolved.

Dora presented with a troubling constellation of symptoms that,
at the outset, like anyone else's, needed to be attributed to a cause.
She had been in poor health most of her life. She'd had episodes of
difficulty breathing starting when she was as young as seven, and as
she grew up, she was plagued with migraines, had difficulty speaking at times, and had a "chronic cough"—a peculiar symptom that
seemed to be somewhat quintessential of hysterics. She was kept at
home throughout most of her young life, schooled by governesses
and tasked with taking care of her family, who were also prone to ill
health, it seemed.

Many scholars at the time would no doubt have thought that Dora's hysteria arose as a culturally acceptable response to emotional
conflict, by which they would have meant, essentially, that her persistent cough was her demure—but increasingly obnoxious—way of
expressing how unhappy she was. Freud's thoughts, however, turned

to the sexual: while Dora was no doubt frustrated that she couldn't receive a real education outside the home, like her brother Otto, Freud
ultimately ascribed her more pervasive depression to frustrations of a
different nature. He first reaches this conclusion when Dora tells him
that after a cousin of hers had appendicitis, she read about the ailment in an encyclopedia, desiring to know what it was. To anyone but
Freud this might be a sign of her curiosity and intelligence. But the
doctor decided that she must have also read about sexual intercourse
in the encyclopedia, and repressed the memory of doing so.

As Dora opens up about her physical symptoms, Freud never
asked what any of her other doctors had said; nor did he himself
probe for a possible organic cause or explanation. Rather, he based
his analysis on a story relayed by Dora's father sometime early in her
treatment. It was this story that became the foundation for Freud's
belief about the girl and her ills. This is interesting, because while the
story was about Dora, it did not come from her. Precisely because it
was delivered to Freud by her father, it was respected as a matter of
fact. It seemed that, during a stay at the lake with a couple who were
friends with Dora's parents, the man—who in the case study went by
Herr K.—made sexual advances toward Dora. Naturally this frightened and confused her.

Herr K. denied any fault when confronted by Dora's father. His
wife, Frau K., who had taken a shine to Dora, further defended him
by implying that Dora "showed an interest in sexual matters and
nothing else." She had probably, said Frau K., misconstrued her inter-
action with Herr K. with something she'd read in a book.

Dora's father told Freud, in no uncertain terms, that he simply
didn't believe his daughter was telling the truth. He refused to break
off his friendship with the couple and felt quite sorry, in particular,
for Frau K.: "Poor woman, she is very unhappy with her husband, of
whom, incidentally, I don't have the highest opinion."

Essentially, Dora's own father sided with the man she had accused of being sexually inappropriate with her because he wanted to
remain on good terms with the man's wife. Even Dora's mother was
an apologist, relaying a story to Dora about how Frau K. had followed
Dora's father into the woods when he had meant to commit suicide,
and convinced him that he must stay alive for his family. Dora did

not believe this story for a second, assuming instead that the two had probably been caught together in the woods, and her father had fabricated a great story of salvation to cover up their tryst.

Despite Dora's pleas, her father held firm. He asked Freud to "please bring her [Dora] around to a better way of thinking"—that is, his way. He did admit, though it wasn't much help, that the entire situation was probably the reason for Dora's "low spirits, irritability and ideas of suicide."

Dora later revealed to Freud that the advance by Herr K. had not been the first: years earlier, when she was just fourteen, he had kissed her quite suddenly upon the lips while they were attending a church festival. She told Freud that it had disgusted her—a reaction that Freud said was most certainly a hysteric one.

"I would without another thought consider anyone a hysteric if a cause for sexual arousal evokes overwhelmingly or exclusively feelings of disgust in her, whether or not she shows somatic symptoms," he wrote in her case study. He called the reaction *affective reversal*. A healthy girl, he wrote, would have felt genital arousal at such an act. The disgust that lingered, morphing into a depression and overall avoidance of Herr K. (or any man who sought only to "engage her in amicable conversation"), seemed to further prove his point.

He also felt that Dora's problems went back a lot further than her forced sexual awakening. They perhaps began when she was just barely of school age, a time when many children discover that they can use illness as a way to get attention from their parents. Dora had carried this tool of manipulation into her young adult life, Freud reasoned, and was once again employing it, but this time as means to get rid of Herr and Frau K., who were taking her parents' attentions away from her. In the case of her father, she was using her illness to create an even more tangible hostility.

As for explaining away her physical symptoms (that pesky cough, for one) Freud thought it was caused by a phantom penis—one that only existed in the fantasies of her mind. Dora, he believed, was having unconscious dick-sucking fantasies that were causing her to have a chronic tickling sensation in her throat, which made her cough.

He noted that this phenomenon was common among his female patients, and that it all stemmed from the suckling at a mother's (or wet-nurse's) breast, which at one time had been associated purely with comfort, safety, and satisfaction. Combine that with Freud's Oedipal theories of father-daughter sexual attraction, and his clinical picture of Dora emerges.

Dora had taken care of her father, who had a chronic illness, for much of her youth, during which time she had become his confidante. She was arguably closer to him than her mother was, as her mother had not exactly been in the wifely way with him for quite some time. Dora's relationship with her father, Freud said, had been shattered by the appearance of his alleged mistress, Frau K., and Freud believed that this disruption was the key event that had precipitated Dora's own ailments.

As it turned out, Dora's story had a somewhat tidy conclusion: several months after she stopped seeing Freud for analysis, she reported back to him that she had gone to visit the K.'s after the death of one of their children, intending to reconcile with them. She had called out Frau K. for sleeping with her father—an accusation the woman did not deny—and gotten Herr K. to admit that he had made sexual advances toward her. She had taken this information back to her father, feeling entirely vindicated.

She was feeling very well after this cathartic meeting until mid-autumn, she said, when she suddenly developed another attack of her symptoms. Freud asked her what had caused it, and she said that she had witnessed a man being run over by a streetcar. The man had been coming toward her on the street, and when he saw her he stopped short, right in the midst of busy traffic.

That man was Herr K. She was, of course, horrified—but would it be a stretch to imagine there was relief in there, too?

She told Freud that she no longer spoke with Frau K. or with her father, and was instead "focused on her studies and had no intention of marrying." (With glib satisfaction, Freud noted at the end of her case study that she did eventually marry.)

⁓⟨⟩

ALTHOUGH I'D READ ABOUT DORA'S case in high school, she would invariably come up again during my freshman year at Sarah Lawrence. When I arrived in the fall of 2009, my housing was an apartment building on Midland Avenue called Hill House that was a solid fifteen-minute walk to campus. I hardly minded, though, because as a freshman it meant I had an apartment with a kitchen, bathrooms, and living spaces. It was co-ed, and three of my five suite-mates were male.

Although Rebecca was my first college friend, and the friendship that ultimately endured once I left, she lived down the hall from me freshman year, and we met through the person I actually shared a room with: a diminutive but fiery girl from Ithaca named Ali. She was an incredibly gifted musician and artist, and despite the fact that she was considerably more outgoing than I was, we quickly hit it off. Almost straightaway, we fell into a routine of huddling together to watch *Bones* every week. She took to comparing me to the titular character, Temperance "Bones" Brennan: a crime-solving forensic pathologist and somewhat socially inept genius who had been kicked around the foster care system (ultimately escaping it). I tried to focus on the more positive aspects of the comparison, though there certainly may have been more than a grain of truth in the less flattering ones.

While I might have been called chatty and personable in high school, I immediately withdrew into myself once I started college. I think my two solid years of psychotherapy beforehand—while ultimately necessary and something I didn't regret at all—may have made me a little *too* cognizant of my defects. Particularly my tendency toward exasperating enthusiasm. So, that first year, I didn't talk much—except by making an occasional attempt to insert some witty retort into the conversation, which I couldn't resist. Instead, I spent most of my social hours observing. I was delighted by my studies, and therefore focused on them, and I devoured my new surroundings. I remember waking up every day and leaping out of bed, wanting to fully experience every single sensation of my days from start to finish. The sound of the boys rustling in their room, searching for socks beneath their alpine piles of laundry. The smell emanating from the apartment of our next-door neighbor, David, who baked the most amazing cookies at one o'clock in the morning. The sound of my shoes slapping wet pavement as I hustled across campus to my first lecture. The acrid taste of the coffee in the dining hall that I learned to tolerate, and the countless early mornings I spent alone, having my breakfast under a large tree as birds chirped above my head and professors lumbered sleepily toward their offices.

This sudden burst of keen interest in every minute of my life was an entirely new experience for me. Even when I inevitably felt bogged down by schoolwork that kept me up late in the library, or endured dance injuries that benched me for a few days, there was never anything that truly discouraged me. I began to feel as though everything was an opportunity, a choice. I felt that I was in complete control of what happened to me.

Those around me—friends and professors—took me for who I wanted to be. Who I was trying so eagerly to become. My intellectual intensity was rewarded and a source of praise from my professors. Perhaps they sensed that I was desperately in need of their praise, or maybe—*just maybe*, they actually meant it.

My adviser was the head of the dance program—Sara Rudner, who had been the muse of the incomparable Twyla Tharp. She was well into her sixties by the time I studied under her, but she was still teaching a full schedule and choreographing with the same passion she had in the 1970s, when she had danced with the likes of Mikhail Baryshnikov and Christopher Janney.

I actually didn't have a very meaningful dance background when I arrived at Sarah Lawrence. I had begun attending dance classes in early childhood, as many little girls do, and had I not had such a nomadic existence, they no doubt would have continued with more consistency. I had the basics down, having continued my lessons sporadically when possible, but I had not been able to develop my skills beyond what repertoire productions of musicals had required of me. And I loved the *art* of dance, though I knew very little about its history. Eager to learn, I loaded up on history and critiquing courses as well as actual dance classes, which took up the majority of my week.

I had no aspirations about becoming a professional dancer, but I did like to envision dances without actually being part of them. Choreography and critique appealed to my auditory and visual senses, and I knew—from learning about the work of Agnes De Mille, who was not regarded as a technically proficient dancer herself, but was certainly lively, and has a beloved place in the canon of dance history—that for a lot of people, that could be enough.

One of the reasons I knew I would never dance professionally, or even as well as the majority of my classmates at the barre, was that I struggled to comprehend the meaning of my body in space. Growing up, I had always been perceived as being "too much," and I had internalized this perception of myself until it became a deeply rooted belief. I later came to understand that it prevented me from being particularly good at moving through the world. I could never escape the notion that I was not wanted, wherever I was. The dance studio was no different. Taking up space, breathing in air, having a place at the barre—I didn't feel like I deserved it. While I hadn't acquired much evidence to the contrary in my life before I arrived at Sarah Lawrence, once I got there, I was imbued with not just permission to be there, but to be alive. I still remember the night I was standing on the sidewalk with one of the girls in my dance class, Rachel, waiting for the shuttle. It was late, and I was tired, and as we were talking about the challenges of our dance curriculum I teared up under that streetlight. I told her that, really, I wasn't a dancer. I had never had consistent training. There were dancers in our class who were already in companies, who had expensive leotards instead of tattered hand me downs.

"I'm not a dancer," I said, expecting Rachel to agree with me. She certainly was a dancer, and one that I had come to admire a lot because not only could she dance, but she could make dances.

She didn't agree with me, though. Instead she laughed, shaking her head of dark curls.

"You love dance, don't you? Even when it's hard?" she asked, her voice the only sound cutting through the night, as if campus and the street had hushed so that I'd hear her clearly.

"Yeah," I said, my mouth curling around a smile that felt too big for my mouth. "I do."

"Look down," she said, "Look at your feet. Look at how you stand."

I looked down at my feet: turned out, first position.

"You are a *dancer!*" she laugh-yelled in that overtired way that always seems a little magical in the dark, cool hours of the night. We giggled as we turned sloppy, joyful pirouettes on the sidewalk in the moonlight.

Not long after that in the relaxed, communal atmosphere of the tiny kitchen of the little apartment in Hill House, I opened up a bit more about my mysterious past with a kind of bitter humor that hit all the right notes among my new liberal artist pals. "It's so raw, so real," one of them mused. "That's what makes it funny!"

I told Rebecca far more specifics about my life than anyone else. After weeks of traipsing back and forth between our apartments on opposite ends of the second-floor hallway, we'd found ourselves kindred spirits. One night, out of earshot of everyone else, I'd told her a bit more about all the people who had been a part of my life, the village that had raised me when my parents had proved unable and, at times, unwilling to do so. Her brow knit in a way I would become familiar with—her endearing, perturbed kind of thoughtfulness—and she said, "You know something, I'm listening to you tell me about all these people, and you're talking about how unique and special they all are for loving you—but what if it's _you_?"

Despite Rebecca's encouraging thought on the matter, as the semester wore on my doubts continued to niggle at me. Bringing up the past I was trying to escape hadn't helped. I began to feel like I couldn't possibly have a future ahead of me any brighter than what I could light myself with the kindling provided to me in the form of scholarship money and bagels stolen from the dining hall. I was constantly afraid that it would all evaporate in the night like a circus soundlessly leaving town.

There were moments when I would sit in the library, staring down the stacks, wondering what I would do if, suddenly, I couldn't be there anymore. What were my options, really? I couldn't just "go home." I couldn't return to the life that I was painstakingly erasing and replacing with each day that passed. I was almost painfully happy at Sarah Lawrence. It wasn't even about the school—it was about who I had become when I set foot there.

When I sensed that my emotions were beginning to get the better of me, I did what any self-respecting academic would do and turned them into a thesis topic. My psychology professor, Elizabeth, was lovely and brilliant: educated at St. Andrews and Oxford, tall, commanding yet kind, with a practical but classy wardrobe. She was everything I wanted to become. From the moment I proposed my topic—Mary Ainsworth and theories of maternal attachment—she seemed to infer that there was far more vested in it than interest.

Elizabeth spoke with a hushed, yet never wavering voice. Combined with the lilt of her accent, this made her a reassuring person to talk with. As it pertained to my proposal on Ainsworth's work, she gently offered that many psychologists took on topics because they were attempting to resolve something from their own psyches.

Likewise, my weekly meetings with Sara, my adviser and dance teacher, began to yield the occasional anecdote from my past— mostly as it pertained to my worries about not being good enough. The pressure to make sure I did everything right all the time wore on me, but I had to harness it and allow it to motivate me. The work I was doing—both academically and on myself—was what I had been aspiring to for as long as I could remember. And I had finally arrived. Still, there was a rigidness that I couldn't seem to shed. A wizened maturity that aged me rather than enlightened me. I had a peculiar heaviness to my nature that I think, at times, unsettled my peers and concerned my mentors.

This rigidness was illustrated most obviously in my dancing— which was restrained and lacking elegance. I didn't like to really try something until I was sure I wouldn't look foolish, and this unwillingness to stumble slowed my progress.

One day in Sara's contemporary class, we were doing some kind of improvisation—which I didn't like, because I had no idea what was expected of me. As I moved my body, torquing it into some slight variation on interesting, I lost my balance and began to fall. Instinct took over and I righted myself, stopping to see if anyone had seen me. Sara had, and she halted the entire class, walking with her small, quick steps across the floor until she was right in my face.

"Did you feel what just happened there?" she said, a wide—but warning—smile spreading across her face.

"I lost my balance, then I corrected—"

She put her hand on my arm. "You let go and something beautiful happened," she whispered, looking me straight in the eye. "Do that more."

AFTER MY FIRST SURGERY, IT was not made clear to me when I would be well again—or if I would ever be well. After conferring with Dr. Paulson and my few close (and unnerved) friends, I decided it was best that I not return to Sarah Lawrence for the spring semester. I would remain in Maine. It didn't hit me right away that what it really meant was that I was never going back—*ever*. I thought I would just return in the fall, even though that meant I'd have to start the year over again, that I would be a year behind. I believed that lie for a long time—until several years after I would have graduated, in fact. I held onto that magical thinking well beyond when it had ceased to serve me, because I was afraid of my own grief.

My life in those first weeks, after the pain returned, was an endless cycle of worry, heating pads, and half-eaten sleeves of saltines. The only things that saved me were journaling and my sessions with Jane—which I had steadily come to resent, because they only seemed to reinforce the idea that something actually was wrong with me. Her practice was in the same town as most of my doctors, a community that was more affluent than the one I'd grown up in. It was more a place we'd visit once a summer as kids to eat overpriced seafood and romp on the beach. My weekly sojourns to her office took me through winding back roads and around mountains that opened up onto a vast, almost breathing sea. I remember how, on particularly awful days, when I felt so bad physically that I wasn't even certain I should have been behind the wheel, I'd look out over that landscape and think: y'know, there are worse places to die. Something about being nestled between the ocean and the mountains made me feel safe, protected. I had once written a poem about the place: *I drove to a place where I felt small and realized I never wanted to feel small at all.*

Returning there out of necessity, to go to the hospital or to see Jane, seemed almost serendipitous. It was as if the universe wanted to protect me. The way my family hadn't. The way no one could.

There were some realities that no one could save me from: mounting medical debt being one. In February 2011, not even six months after I'd been in the hospital in New York, I got the first of what would be hundreds of calls from a collection agency. I had no idea what to do. I had put those first payments onto the one credit card I had, noting in my journal that "every single time I use it I feel like I'm destined to end up $100,000 in debt," though at the time, it only had a $600 balance. Still, when you're dirt poor, not bringing in any income, and now you owe people money, $600 might as well be $100,000. The calls kept coming, and I kept crying and trying to pay what I could, but by the end of the year I had racked up several thousand dollars in medical debt, a trend that would continue for the next five or so years.

All of this, and I still didn't even really understand what I was dealing with. Was this thing, this endometriosis, supposed to make me feel this bad? That didn't seem reasonable. And besides, when Dr. Paulson had mentioned it, she'd merely done so as if it were some incidental finding. Like when I'd had that MRI in high school and they'd told me I had low-lying cerebellar tonsils. It didn't really mean anything. Endometriosis couldn't be serious, because if it was, wouldn't she have said so? Wouldn't she have told me what to do? Or recommended another doctor, or prescribed me a medication? I didn't even really understand what it was, but I trusted that it wasn't anything that mattered, because Dr. Paulson, and my regular doctor, and anyone else I ever mentioned it to in passing, acted like it didn't. Oddly enough, the only thing that seemed to reassure me was that I was still getting periods, although they were, as ever, erratic. I took that as a sign that at the very least I wasn't anorexic, like my mother. I reasoned I wouldn't be having a period if I was, conveniently ignoring the fact that my mother's illness had never exactly been accurately reflected by her menstrual cycle (me being the proof).

There was something oddly comforting about the fact that when I did get a period, it seemed to be just as bad as always. I bled all over the place per usual. I did, however, find it much harder to tolerate the cramps mostly because I was exhausted to begin with, and probably more than a little anemic.

Jane had her own theories to posit as a psychologist: namely, that perhaps we needed to consider the possibility that all of this stemmed from some emotional holding tank. At first this was a theory I refused to acknowledge on principle, but when I considered it rationally, it didn't seem *that* far-fetched: we could argue that everyone has some Dark Secret From Their Past that gives them insomnia and the occasional anxiety-induced stomachache.

And in fact, what was once termed *hysteria* has evolved into what is now called *conversion disorder*, where a neurological symptom develops for which there is no physiological explanation or known organic cause. That doesn't mean it isn't real, though: the patient is not malingering or putting on his or her symptom; it occurs unconsciously and is not under the person's conscious control. Although conversion disorder may share some features with its hysterical progenitor, its presentation and diagnostic criteria are actually quite specific. One of its most prominent features is that the patient does not seem very worried about the symptom (exhibiting *la belle indifférence*)—and it typically is just one symptom, usually of neurologic origin. It may manifest as something like a repetitive jerking motion, a loss of a sense (vision or smell), or paralysis of a limb. If the episodes recur, however, that one symptom might change, or move to a new location. True conversion disorder is actually very rare: the National Organization for Rare Disorders puts its incidence rate at less than 25 cases per 100,000 people.

There are other, more frequently encountered descendants of hysteria, though: hypochondria, malingering, and somatization disorders, for instance. While people often regard somatization disorder as being "all in the head," by definition it involves very real physical symptoms, which the patient is not faking. The disorder is actually less about whatever the physical symptoms may be (which can vary across multiple body systems, progress through them, or occur concurrently) and more about how the person is responding to them. While the patient with conversion disorder may appear totally unconcerned by the fact that they've suddenly lost their vision, a person with somatization disorder may be extremely distressed by a number of physical ailments, which are often quite vague and for which no apparent cause is found when imaging, bloodwork, or even surgical procedures are undertaken. It still does not mean that the symptoms aren't real and capable of causing distress. It may be that, as a result of general disposition and personality, underlying depression or an anxiety disorder, or even cultural and anthropological influences that shape how we view the sick, some patients are much more sensitive than others to the experience of being unwell. Some research suggests there are people who happen to be extremely aware of their normal bodily processes, to the point where normal functions actually feel abnormal. Thus, they experience a constant barrage of unnerving feelings that, in reality, are just their bodies doing what bodies do.

Contrary to what it may sound like, I did not immediately reject the mind-body theory to explain my symptoms. In fact, I'd been considering it long before any doctor suggested it. When I went back through emails and social media posts from the weeks right before I got sick, I realized there had been some experiences that could have been considered prodromal—except that I'd readily written them off as stress.

By the time I reached Sarah Lawrence, I had been working through my myriad emotional traumas with Jane for a couple of years. The whole reason I'd made a beeline for her office after getting emancipated was that I wanted to figure out how screwed up I was and do something about it. I didn't have any illusions about my mental health: I figured I had probably been clinically depressed since my preteen years, and was demonstrably anxiety-ridden long before that. I was completely ready and willing to admit that, just like almost anyone else at one time or another, I had physical symptoms that were attributable to being in a state of emotional stress. I understood the cause-and-effect relationship even as a kid—I have always assumed it was an acquired skill because I had to be hypervigilant about what the adults around me were feeling. That wasn't necessarily an easy task, because they could be quite volatile. I had to be able to make quick, rational analysis of their moods so I could predict their behavior. I suppose it was only natural that, eventually, I'd come to practice the same kind of objective self-assessment on myself.

In the context of psychotherapy, I found this particularly helpful, but I've often wondered if Jane ever felt like I was trying to do her job. Of course, even if I had wanted to, I never could have truly given myself that kind of unbiased appraisal, and I knew that. I knew I couldn't do the work I needed to do alone, and that's why I'd sought Jane out in the first place, why I kept showing up in her office week after week, season after season, year after year. I wasn't sure the work would ever be done, but by the time I was ready to leave for college, I felt like I had made a respectable amount of progress. At the very least, I had faced the crucible of my dysfunction head-on and come away with a tidy list of my foibles and shortcomings—none of which seemed particularly exceptional. Not just in the context of my upbringing, but for most adult humans I knew in general. The things I'd started to work on, and I assumed would continue to work on indefinitely, seemed to me like garden-variety emotional quibbles: I had a hard time trusting people, I had a fair amount of social awkwardness (which typically manifested in a quickly fatiguing degree of loquaciousness), and I probably had a tad more insecurity than other girls my age. The only real eccentricities, that seemed unique to me and my situation were my vomiting phobia (which drunk college roommates would provide exposure therapy for in due time) and the push-pull dynamic I tended to form with older, maternal women, which could be almost concussive in its intensity.

Although I may not have always known exactly what it was I needed to do to "work on" these parts of myself, I was always aware that they were there. If they popped up, I'd hear Jane's voice in my head asking me if they were needed, or if they were old conditioned responses that weren't serving me anymore. Figuring out the answer to that question wasn't something that I was immediately good at, but, as with many things in life, it got easier with practice. Where this became particularly relevant was in those moments when I had a very strong emotional response to something—strong enough to be felt throughout my body.

When I first got sick and reviewed how I was feeling, I expected to be able to link my symptoms to an obvious, rational cause—likely a stressful one. Upon closer inspection, I had to admit that how I felt was not the usual way stress manifested inside of my body. The pain, the nausea, the utter exhaustion: it was all different—and in a number of key ways.

For one thing, the pain was extremely specific. The vague stomach and chest pain that came from panic and anxiety were nothing like the persistent, pulsing ache that seemed to have taken up residence between my midriff, hip bone, and lower back. The dizziness and nausea that came from nerves was nothing like the sudden, breathtaking nausea that overtook me after just a few bites of food. I would often still be in want of food, but, simultaneously, somehow also be on the verge of vomiting. At night, the nausea would get so bad that I would lie half-awake on the bathroom floor holding my breath, because even the exertion of my diaphragm and lungs seemed to make it worse.

And the exhaustion was like nothing I had ever experienced in my life. I had been dancing for six or seven hours a day at Sarah Lawrence. I had worked summer jobs where I was lugging laundry up and down stairs all day, enduring grueling rehearsal schedules, and hiking through the woods of Maine as a meter-reader. I knew what it felt like to come home at the end of a long day with burning muscles and eyes that couldn't stay open.

I also became unusually prone to spilling things, or knocking things over, or running into walls. I had experienced such an epiphany about my body in space through dance—not being able to orient myself was startling and maddeningly disappointing. Further, it just didn't make sense. I had lost nearly fifty pounds, and was whittled down to near nothing. How was it that, being so small, I was more ungainly and uncoordinated than I had been when I had taken up more space?

Surely some of my struggles were simply from losing so much weight. But why had I lost it? Why couldn't I eat? Why was I in pain? Why was I still bleeding as though my uterus were a bottomless pool of blood?

The pain was real and it was demanding. While Jane sipped her tea and nodded a lot, I retraced the weeks leading up to when I had left Sarah Lawrence. I tried to work out why and how and when the pain actually started. I began telling her about when I was admitted to the hospital the first time, then the second. How I had been in the position of having to explain that no, in fact, there was no one that they could call for me.

She perked up at this, realizing that in those hours of need I had been totally alone. The hospital was not obligated to call my parents. They did not call anyone. This seemed to unsettle her, and in a very uncharacteristic lapse into her own psyche, she said, to herself mostly, "When my daughter was in the hospital they called me in the middle of the night. They wouldn't do a thing without talking to her mother first . . ." As quickly as this new understanding had shadowed her face, it disappeared, replaced by her glassy-eyed professionalism. But I never forgot it. Because, as I watched that flicker of compassion fall across her face, I felt some for myself—if only fleetingly.

At the time, I was annoyed with her. I wrote a good paragraph in my journal about how irked I'd been that she'd become a three-dimensional person, even briefly. That wasn't what she got paid for— she didn't get paid to have *feelings*! She got paid to witness *me* having feelings!

"Jane doesn't try to make my life worse," I wrote, as though my pen had mightily heaved a sigh. "She just does."

THE NEXT DAY, I WENT to see a new doctor, in a new office, in a new town, for a second opinion. Actually, to be precise, he was like the fifth or sixth doctor I'd seen by that point. I was actually being sent to him because my regular doctor had felt a lump in my lower back that she wanted him to look at.

Dr. Wagstaff was of dad-age and had the most friendly office staff I've ever encountered—then or since. I got the feeling that his receptionist hated leaving for lunch, lest she miss out on their witty repartee. I was ushered into an exam room, and he popped in moments later—a remarkably short wait time. He greeted me in a friendly, fatherly tone and proceeded to palpate a lump in my lower back.

"Lipoma," he shrugged. "Not to be worried about." He squinted at my record, then sat back in his chair. "But this . . . tell me about this pain you've been having. And the weight loss. And, well," he said, flipping a page over, "everything else."

So, I did. And when he inquired with genuine curiosity whether or not I had family to fall back on, I tried to make light of the situation by throwing in the anecdote about living within an unusual proximity to Cass's staircase.

"So, basically, you're Harry Potter—but with a lot of Anne Hathaway going on," he said, gesturing vaguely to my overall appearance. I laughed when I wanted to cringe, because that was pretty much what I'd been taught about dealing with men in any situation, but certainly in those where I was clearly not the one in power.

Though he thought the lipoma wasn't anything to bother with, Dr. Wagstaff could see that I was troubled by the other symptoms. He was more troubled by my life story, though, and wondered aloud— much to my horror—if my psyche was to blame. I don't think he meant to be problematic when he posited this aloud to me, but he didn't do so with very much tact.

"You were probably molested as a child and this is just your body's way of trying to handle it," he said as he made a note on my chart. As though it were a completely reasonable thing to say. I raised an eyebrow in contempt—surely the seat of my emotional discontent would not sequester itself to a single organ. And even if it had, perhaps this was not the time or the place to bring it up. Certainly not quite so casually.

Even if he believed I had psychosomatic problems, he did order some tests. First, he wanted to rule out some kind of intestinal parasite, so he prescribed me more antibiotics. He wasn't entirely convinced it would help, but at the very least it was one more thing we could definitively rule out.

He couldn't promise that he'd be able to help me, regardless of what the tests said. He stood as he ripped a slip from his prescription pad and handed it to me. "Your problem is complicated," he said simply. "Just like *you*."

To no one's surprise, the antibiotics didn't help. In fact, they made me feel a lot worse. Antibiotics, notorious for causing diarrhea, didn't help me keep weight on, and I grew wearier and wearier as the weeks went by.

When I went to my next session with Jane, I told her what Dr. Wagstaff had said: that my problem was complicated and that I was complicated. She responded by admitting that she, too, at times, had wondered if she could truly help me. This caught me completely off-guard, and though it was humiliating to find myself doing so, I immediately began to cry. It wasn't "close up on Meryl Streep's face" crying, either. It was "I'm five years old and my life is hard" crying.

I wheezed and snotted until I collapsed in on myself, and on her stiff couch, because I finally realized that maybe all of this had been my fault. Maybe I had done something that I shouldn't have done, or not done something that I should have done, and it had caused this. The harder I cried, the more convinced I became that it was the truth.

"I did this!" I announced, somewhat agog, and to no one in particular. "I made this happen—it was my fault, wasn't it?" I buried my face between the pillows, not even bothering with tissues, which I did not feel I deserved.

"No," she said quietly, but firmly. I heard her put down her pen and notepad. She cleared her throat, and though I couldn't see her face, I heard something in her voice that made me pause and listen. "It wasn't your fault. This isn't your fault."

DESPITE HAVING BEEN ON ANTIBIOTICS, I came down with a horrific bout of bronchitis in the weeks that followed, so I didn't go to my next appointment with Jane or anyone else. I did, however, take my first job since I'd left school: a professional theater company I'd worked with my senior year of high school offered me a part in its spring show. I took it, desperate for the money—and for a chance to attempt to get back a semblance of the life I'd had before. Problems arose, mostly to do with my period. In order to avoid bleeding through my costumes, I wore bike shorts with two or three overnight Maxi Pads stuck in them, which felt like a diaper, but kept me from unwittingly inserting bloodshed into a scene in which it had not been scripted. The bleeding had gotten even worse since I'd gone off the birth control pill I had been taking, which the pharmaceutical company had suddenly stopped manufacturing. I couldn't afford any of the other ones.

It was also during this time that I remembered that I'd have to drive to Sarah Lawrence to get all of my things from the dorm Rebecca and I had been sharing. Cass said she'd drive me, knowing that it would be both physically uncomfortable and emotionally precarious for me to go alone. When we arrived, I hugged Rebecca for a long time. All my old friends came to help us load up Cass's truck with my things.

I had considered staying on campus long enough to visit with everyone. I could explain what had happened, go see my professors. But I was overcome with grief, the certitude that I would never come back, and it was crashing down on me as I watched all the pieces of me being stowed away in boxes—and not for the first time in my life. I'd moved so much over the past eight years that this shouldn't have fazed me, but it felt different. I had wanted, more than anything, to be there. The best year of my life had been spent toiling around that campus, laughing until I cried late at night, coming back from the city on the Metro-North to Yonkers, beginning to figure out who I was and what I wanted to do with my life among some of the most vibrant and intelligent people I'd ever known. To be standing there, watching my entire life be packed up, felt like a terrible mistake. I swallowed down the urge to cry out, "No! Put it back! This is all wrong, I can still be here, I still want to be here!"

But it didn't matter. It never had. What was happening within me was indifferent to the life that I wanted, that I'd worked so hard for. It watched, as my friends did, as I slunk into Cass's truck and we drove away, back to Maine, all my chances lost.

CHAPTER 6

The patient is always the ultimate source of knowledge.

—Philip Bonnet, quoted in Terry R. Bard,
Medical Ethics in Practice

NOÉMIE ELHADAD IS AN ASSOCIATE professor of biomedical informatics at Columbia University, a researcher, and an endometriosis patient. Five years after I was diagnosed with endometriosis myself, I would speak at the Endometriosis Foundation of America's annual medical conference, which is where I met Noémie. On a subsequent trip to New York City, I arranged to meet up with her at a café in Columbus Circle, arriving covered in a sheen of sweat and regret after greatly overestimating how many blocks I could reasonably walk before I got nauseated. I was a little late, but from the beginning Noémie was generous not just with her time, but with her kindness.

We sat at a table near the back, hoping to keep the noise of the bustling café from cutting through my recording of our conversation. Two things struck me about Noémie within the first five minutes of our interview: she's brilliant and pleasant, in equal measure, which is to say, exceptionally so. In my dealings with those in the upper echelons of academia, I have often found that the two are inversely proportional. So Noémie's conversational, genuine, and witty demeanor was a welcome reprieve, not only from the scholarly grind I'd been in, but from the nauseated and exhausted state I was in when we met.

She spoke with the soft remnants of a French accent, and as soon became clear, it was as a young girl in France that her endometriosis began. The very fact that she had begun her journey with the disease so young was indicative of the fact that she had not grown up in the United States, but in Europe, where there seems to be a greater awareness of the condition, not to mention more equitable access to care.

"I was diagnosed at age fourteen without any problem," she said. "There was not even a search for a diagnosis. It was like, 'Thirteen, first period, crappy for like six months,' and at fourteen, it was like, 'Yup, that's what you have.'"

"It's not like it helped me to have known it earlier," Noémie admitted, pointing out that in her case, despite having a name for her suffering and being started on the familiar course of treatments— including "a few crappy years" of Lupron—knowing sooner didn't seem to stall the progression of the disease.

As she got older, she began to worry about her fertility. But she experienced firsthand, and debunked firsthand, two of the most prevalent myths about endometriosis: that she wouldn't be able to get pregnant (she did), and that pregnancy would cure her endo (it didn't). In fact, Noémie noted, it was a bit jarring for her to begin menstruating again while she was still breastfeeding her daughter—a time during which most women experience a normal bout of amenorrhea that's mediated by lactation. Noémie's menstrual cycle returned just one month after she gave birth. So did her endo symptoms.

As she recounted this story, we both laughed a bit. At the time, it felt like we were just throwing our hands up at the absurdity of it, but months later, as I listened to the tape of the interview, I can hear the sadness just below. We shared a kind of resolution to pessimism, and she openly admitted to that throughout our conversation.

Noémie channeled her frustration, however, seamlessly into her work. Her current research project at Columbia, the development of a tracking app called Phendo, was her attempt to quantify the unquantifiable, not only for herself, but for the collective. For science, and for patients.

One thing that's missing from our understanding of endometriosis at every level, as Noémie pointed out, is its phenotype. For a disease like endo, a phenotype is the set of characteristics that can be observed: symptoms, test results, and microscopic evidence from tissue samplings, for example. Noémie and her team developed Phendo in the hope that they would be able to utilize a "citizen science" initiative to gather information about endo patients' experiences, histology, and biomarkers. Unlike most tracking apps of its kind, it isn't menstruation-centric, because endometriosis, Noémie believes, is not a menstruation-specific disease. "Many women in our online surveys are on hormonal treatments and have no period at all, but symptoms are still present. It's not about the periods anymore, especially for women who have lived with endo for a while," she later told me in an email, after Phendo had launched for Apple devices.

Noémie's inclination to broaden the scope of discussion and research around endometriosis is important—in part because calling it a "female disease," or a "period problem," excludes entire groups of people who may have endometriosis but do not identify as female. Ren, for example, who is in his twenties, has stopped menstruating at this point in his transition because of hormone replacement therapy. But when he was still getting periods, which he recalls as being heavy and painful, doctors were reluctant to even consider endometriosis: they felt the hormone therapy required to facilitate his female-to-male transition should have "cleared it up." When Ren was no longer bleeding, however, he still experienced severe, chronic pain. When he started researching his symptoms, endometriosis came up as a possibility. One that, because of how endometriosis is framed as a menstruation-dependent ailment, was difficult for him to reckon with. "Everything online talks about it as a woman's disease, and I am a transgender man," Ren told me. "So it feels very dehumanizing to read resources about it. And it's already difficult enough to deal with."

As it turns out, Ren does have endometriosis: it was surgically confirmed. Such confirmation is routinely difficult even for women to obtain, but as a trans individual, Ren found it especially difficult to access reproductive health care. "Now that I've been physically transitioning for a long time," he said, "it's made the process awkward and uncomfortable at best. Walking into or calling the OB/GYN always leads to a lot of scrutiny, confusion, or uncomfortable assumptions and interactions." One time, for example, a nurse called and asked for Ann (his birth name)—and then asked if he was her husband.

Saying that endometriosis (like hysteria before it) is a disease exclusive to women, or even of uteruses, isn't just noninclusive—it's not true. Endometriosis has been found in men. Take this clinical portrait: an eighty-five-year-old man had an endometrioma in his abdomen, and for ten years, it was believed to be a carcinoma of the prostate. When they studied this patient's chromosomes, he was phenotypically male, and, as it turned out, he did in fact have prostate cancer. But he also had an endometrioma that was independent of the cancer.

Another more recent case involved a fifty-two-year-old man who came to the emergency room with stabbing pain in his lower abdomen and pelvis which had been ongoing for about three weeks. He had a history of advanced liver disease and had had several surgeries to fix an inguinal hernia over the past two years. When a laparotomy was performed, a cystic mass was found attached to his bladder. The pathology revealed a lesion of thick, smooth muscle fibers with estrogen and progesterone receptors—consistent with endometriosis.

In both cases, the foremost question is: If endometriosis is supposed to be displaced uterine tissue, then how the hell does it wind up inside someone with no uterus?

One explanation might be found during fetal development. At around seven weeks, the reproductive systems of all fetuses look about the same. At this point, it could go either way: the fetus could develop male sex organs or female sex organs. They have both Wolffian ducts (male) and Müllerian ducts (female). Only one set of ducts will remain, and that's determined by the interplay of genetics (X and Y chromosomes) and hormones.

We know that this process of sexual differentiation doesn't always go off without a hitch: sometimes it's incomplete, and a baby is born intersex, meaning that the baby has both kinds of chromosomes and reproductive organs. Sometimes male babies can be born androgen-sensitive, with more biologically female development, or females can be born with congenital adrenal hyperplasia, meaning that they produce too much cortisol, which behaves similarly to testosterone.

There are also cases where prolonged estrogen therapy—like in the case of prostate cancer—seems to lead to the finding of endometriosis in male patients. In a case from Japan, a sixty-nine-year-old man who had been undergoing hormone therapy for nine years to treat prostate cancer developed a sizable endometrial lesion in the structures surrounding the testes. His doctors hypothesized that the estrogen therapy had encouraged cells to undergo both *metaplasia* (meaning they changed type) and *hyperplasia* (meaning the therapy encouraged an increase in stromal cells).

There are at least six other reports in current literature of endometriosis in male patients undergoing long-term estrogen therapy for prostate cancer, including one man who was just twenty-seven years old. Six may not sound like a lot, but it's noteworthy that in all six cases, endometriosis was accurately diagnosed, even when other conditions, such as cancer, were also present and could have confounded the diagnostic process. From the discussions of these studies, it appears that these men saw a resolution in symptoms attributable to endometriomas through surgery or the removal of estrogen therapy (they may have had lingering symptoms attributable to cancer or its treatment, of course). But the fact that they saw any improvement at all makes sense, because men are not estrogen-dependent creatures by nature. Women, however, do not have it quite so easy, starting from the moment they begin to express that they are in pain. Especially pain related to their periods.

I FIRST GOT MY PERIOD on Thanksgiving day when I was twelve and a half, which was more or less the developed world average at the time for menarche. I was ripped, because Thanksgiving was the one day of the year that I was allowed to eat unfettered. Despite Mum's disapproving glares, she could do nothing about it as I shoveled pie into my face. My father, too, enjoyed the holiday for this reason. You can only imagine my dismay when, by midmorning, before the food was even out of the oven, I found myself relegated to the bathroom with diarrhea. I was shaking from cramps and had a deep soreness in my upper thighs that almost felt like pulled muscles, except somehow deeper.

The cramping wasn't unusual; I often woke up in the middle of the night with similar symptoms. I would awaken from a dead sleep and sit shaking violently in the bathroom for hours late at night, my legs so wobbly beneath me that when I finally dragged myself back to bed, I'd have to push my knees against the mattress. This all being what robust New Englanders would call a "gut's ache," I tried not to complain about it.

In hindsight, the somewhat cyclical nature of these spells may also have been a harbinger of what was to come once I started menstruating. The same symptoms afflicted me at various points in my hormonal cycle and, in fact, they are an extremely common, shared experience among endometriosis patients. Painful bowel movements are not a symptom that can easily go unnoticed, but it certainly isn't widely discussed.

Since Mum and I were the only people not enjoying the Thanksgiving meal, she was the only one available to check on me. As upset as I was, and as uncomfortable as that made her, I always thought she might have been glad I'd given her a reason to leave the table. All my life I'd hoped, I suppose, that if it came down to food and me, she would not consider me the more odious to endure.

My mother's anorexia meant that she had no menstrual map to give me. As an adult, I would look back and realize that even if she had been menstruating, she knew very little about her own body and wouldn't have had much to offer me. Even if she had had any sentimentality about the clunky yet endearing bonding mothers and daughters generally partake in, she just didn't know enough about herself, emotionally or physiologically, to guide me.

Even without guidance, I was a keen observer, and I figured out the nuances of my cycle fairly quickly: my periods were essentially regular, but extremely heavy. Often they were painful enough for me to want to miss school—which was the first of many subconscious triggers that something wasn't right. I had suffered some substantial illnesses and injuries, and never once had I wanted to miss school on account of them. To the contrary, the worse I felt, the more I needed school to lift my spirits. It was my entire network of love and support, not to mention food. But my periods, with their dizzying fatigue, nausea, and pain, seemed to be the one thing that could put my life on pause.

Once I had left home and was spending my teenage years hopping from couch to couch, my relationship to my period became even more fraught. I knew I had a tendency to bleed through my clothes at night, and the harrowing prospect of bleeding onto the sheets or couches that people were so kindly letting me sleep on made me lie awake in fear many nights. It seemed that no matter how many pads I wore, I'd always end up with blood pouring out of me, either on bed linens or the middle of the bathroom floor.

I tried valiantly to use tampons, but found them gasp-inducing, edge-of-sink-gripping painful. For many reasons, they would have been my preference—not least of all to end the locker room jeering I got for wearing pads. Still, no matter what I did, tampons would cause my entire pelvis to ache, as though the menstrual cramps were echoing, or the tampon a divining rod for pain.

So, I stuck to pads. Or, rather, they stuck to me and everything else. I have, on more than one occasion, retrieved a notebook from my purse during a meeting only to find a panty-liner stuck to it. The foibles of needing to be ever-ready.

Despite the fact that I suspected my periods might not be normal, I admitted that I didn't really know what normal was. I reasoned that I just needed to toughen up about it, and composed rather eloquent and long Freudian explanations, writing in my journals that my periods were probably normal, but that my perception of them was skewed because I had not had a mother to put them into the grander context of my blossoming womanhood. In fact, she had gone so far as to instill in me a certain fear of my own body at an early age.

Regardless, I have since discovered that the widely held belief that a normal menstrual cycle must be twenty-eight days, and that ovulation will occur mid-cycle around or on day fourteen, is not necessarily true. The study that provided the touted twenty-eight-day cycle meant it as an average. In fact, no woman in the study actually had a twenty-eight-day cycle. They all had cycles longer or shorter than twenty-eight days.

These variations exist not only from woman to woman, but even within the same woman throughout the course of her life. A thirteen-year-old girl who has only just started menstruating may not be ovulating at all. Anovulatory cycles, where a woman has a period without ovulating at mid-cycle, can be normal, depending on the age of the woman's menstrual life. But they can also be a sign of subfertility: a young teenager who is not ovulating would not be cause for concern, whereas an otherwise healthy woman in her early thirties should be ovulating quite regularly.

For much of human history, females of the species were locked into near-constant cycles of pregnancy and breastfeeding. The act of breastfeeding suppresses ovulation and menstruation. This was kind of the nicest thing that evolution did for women of the ancient world, because it meant they wouldn't immediately get pregnant while their newborn babies were still entirely dependent on them. Generally, by the time breastfeeding ceased, it meant that a child had (1) survived infancy, and (2) possessed enough independence from mom that she could become busy with a new baby and the child wouldn't die from her negligence.

When a woman breastfeeds, the suckling of the baby is actually what signals her body to start ovulating again. In the first few months of life, the intensity of the baby's suckling action portrays desperation: without the mother at this point, the baby would die. As the baby gets older and enters toddlerhood, the amount of breastfeeding and the intensity of suckling gradually begin to ease off as the child gains more independence. When the suckling lessens, and eventually disappears, it signals the mother's body that it would be okay to get pregnant again.

The caveat? Research has indicated that this is really only protective for about the first six months postpartum. Some women certainly experience lactational amenorrhea for longer, but it's not a sure thing. And these findings are pretty recent—only within the past thirty years. You can imagine that, at the turn of the century and before, women would have struggled to understand their fertility in the best of times, but the fear of getting pregnant so soon after giving birth was very real—in part because childbirth was, for most of history, a fairly dangerous, if not fatal, affair.

IRVINE LOUDON, WHO PUBLISHED A paper on maternal mortality throughout the eighteenth century in 1986, referred to his research

as the study of "a deep, dark and continuous stream of mortality."
Women who died in childbirth either had complications during de-
livery, such as hemorrhaging, or complications after, such as puer-
peral fever. The latter was called "childbed fever," because women
who had just delivered babies in "lying-in hospitals" seemed particularly vulnerable to it. The disease was actually sepsis, a potentially
life-threatening infection of the blood, and it was caused by the very
doctors who treated the women in hospital.

At that point in history, doctors were kind of jacks-of-all-trades:
they delivered babies, treated the sick and injured, and conducted autopsies when necessary. The problem was, they weren't washing their
hands in between. So, a doctor might be conducting an autopsy and
be called away to help deliver a baby. This was before germ theory,
so it never occurred to a doctor to wash up beforehand. Essentially,
doctors were transmitting any and all of the diseases or infections
they encountered in their previous patients (living or dead) to new
mothers and their babies.

When women began dying from sepsis in London hospitals at
a faster clip than women who delivered at home with midwives, a
few pioneering physicians began to investigate (including Dr. Oliver
Wendell Holmes, known best for his poetry, but who was also an accomplished physician). Once medical science discovered and began
to actively crusade against transmissible infection, childbed fever all
but evaporated. But there were still risks to childbirth, many of which
were silent and pernicious.

Eclampsia, a dangerous rise in blood pressure, can cause fatal seizures after a baby is born and may come on quite suddenly.
The youngest daughter of the Crawley family on the beloved period
drama *Downton Abbey* died of this when the two male doctors who
were charged with treating her couldn't agree on her course of treatment: a storyline that, unfortunately, is based on fact.

Of course, for the vast majority of human history, women gave
birth virtually anywhere but in a hospital: at home, at work in the
fields, in a hut or a cave—and certainly these places weren't the most
sterile and safe environments. Yet humankind persisted.

Just as childbirth can endanger a woman's life, so, too, can menstruation. Women today have nearly four times as many periods in

their lifetimes as their ancestors did—around 450 to 500. It might seem like an extremely high number, but consider the following: if a woman begins to menstruate at age twelve and ceases to menstruate at age fifty (averages that are hypothetically perfect but nonexistent in practice on both ends), and she has one period per month during that time, she'll have had 456 periods in her lifetime. Factor in one pregnancy, where her periods would be absent for at least 9 months, or maybe a year if she breastfeeds on demand, and she'd only be down 12 to 15 periods. So even two or three pregnancies would only save her maybe 50 periods in her lifetime. That's still about 400 periods.

Our ancestors didn't have to confront these numbers, because they rarely lived into what we now consider to be middle age. The high end of their life expectancy topped out long before menstruation begins to taper off as women of the modern age enter perimenopause in their early fifties. The historical trend for menarche, meanwhile, has slunk downward. It wasn't unheard of for young women of the *Downton Abbey* era to not begin menstruating until the age of fifteen or sixteen. A woman would likely only have a few years of her "monthlies" before she would marry and begin to have children. The reasons for the declining age at menarche are not yet fully understood, but if you can imagine it—diet, environment, genetics, plastic—someone, somewhere, has likely implicated it.

Today, with menarche happening at age twelve, on average, and women choosing various methods to delay childbearing well into their twenties and thirties (or even longer!), women are having a lot of periods. And not only are they starting them earlier, but they're having them longer (well into their forties and early fifties) largely because they are simply living longer.

The big question is, do women need to menstruate so long? Other than to precipitate childbearing, does menstruation actually have any other purpose? Once a woman completes her childbearing, say, in her late thirties, can she safely stop menstruating? Can a young woman who wishes to delay childbearing for a decade, or indefinitely, use the various methods of hormonal contraception available to her to never have a period?

Dr. Melanie Marin, one of the top gynecologic surgeons in New York, thinks she can—and in fact, that she should. Particularly if she

has debilitating premenstrual symptoms or a condition like endometriosis that makes having a period excruciatingly painful.

DR. MARIN ARRIVED TO MEET me in a café on the Upper West Side
on her bicycle. She shook her neatly cropped blonde hair, a bit askew
from her helmet, out of her eyes as she sat down. Dr. Marin struck me
as being a serious, but not unfriendly, woman in her early forties with
a verbal acuity mirroring the precision required of a surgeon. She's
affiliated with a group of doctors in New York but has surgical and
admitting privileges at Mount Sinai, where she performs surgeries
and oversees the work of her many residents.

Dr. Marin was a young resident at Columbia during a decade
when the crusade for laparoscopic gynecological surgery informed
her education, and certainly it influenced her career as a surgeon.
These methods are still doubted in the setting of grand rounds, but
when it comes to time on the table versus time in recovery, Dr. Marin
thinks the answer is pretty clear: do what's best for the patient.

I was eager to hear from a female physician on the subject of
endometriosis and reproductive health, because even the most as-
tute and competent male physician is still missing that experiential
component of the menstrual cycle that breeds empathy. Although
I acknowledge that physicians of any gender have to put limits on
their empathy—too heavy a dose of it can greatly compromise their
work—I also think that it has a place in the exam room. That being
said, I personally have experienced a lack of empathy from both male
and female physicians around menstruation: women who haven't had
bad periods can't empathize any better with me than men who have
never menstruated.

Recent research from *JAMA Internal Medicine* revealed that
patients have better outcomes when they're treated by female physicians, including being less likely to die. This study, and ones like
it, chalk it all up to differences in how men and women approach
and practice medicine. Female doctors are more likely to encourage
and prescribe preventative care measures and to use more patient-
centered communication techniques. They also seem to have a better handle on what one would call "bedside manner." But medicine

on the whole is still a male-dominated profession: women make up just a third of all doctors in the United States. And certainly education, personality, motivation, resources, location, and many other socioeconomic factors that have nothing to do with gender account for how a particular physician practices. By and large, though, it does seem that much of what we consider traditional thought in medicine stems from its roots as a male-led vocation.

The more physicians and patients I talked to, the more I began to realize that while there are some overarching patriarchal themes, they aren't solely perpetuated by men. Women do it too: every time a mother tells her daughter that bad cramps are just a part of life, or just part of being a woman, she's reinforcing something she's come to understand as fact.

Dr. Marin would beg to differ—on the nature of menstruation, not the patriarchy. Regarding the latter, as we stood to depart at the end of our interview, she glanced down at my notepad where I'd scribbled something about the patriarchy of medicine. She pointed to it and just gave me a simple, but bold and resounding, "*Yes.*"

"I think perhaps my biggest take as a woman is that I have so many people come to me who are willing to tolerate so much, or they have tolerated so much," Dr. Marin began in our discussion of female pain. "Either because no one was willing to listen to them, or just because they thought it was normal, or that was the price of being a woman—that they don't have to tolerate."

Although I presumed that she doesn't have endometriosis herself and told her as much, she added, "I have no idea if I have endometriosis or not. But I always had horrible cramps. With the heating pad on my back, lying on the couch and crying. Heavy periods. Once I realized I didn't have to have a period, I never had a period again."

I actually felt myself staring at her, unsure if I'd heard her correctly. She then went on to say that she hasn't had a period in twenty years. Her menstrual cycle impacted her life so negatively that she—in what I can only describe as enviable pragmatism—took control by using a mix of continuous hormonal birth control options to permanently suppress her period, except for when she wanted to become pregnant.

"You don't have to have a period, ever," she told me unflinchingly. "You should never have a period, unless you're trying to get pregnant. And even then, maybe not. You don't have to have a period. You don't have to have cramps. You don't have to bleed. You don't have to. You ought not to."

She's never looked back, and when it comes to her patients— many of whom are debilitated by their periods because of endometriosis or fibroids—she recommends the same path. It's not uncommon for women to balk at the suggestion: many have asserted that not having a period would feel "unnatural." Dr. Marin acknowledges this, but counters, "We don't know what it means for periods to be 'natural.'"

Dr. Marin, and others, have suggested that the idea that menstruation is the only natural course for a woman is outdated. "People think it's not natural not to bleed—well, it's not natural *to* bleed," she said. "Until the past century or so, women couldn't control their own fertility. For most of human history, monthly periods for thirty or forty years were not the norm. It's only in the past eighty to one hundred years that women have had enough control over their fertility that they've had periods for so long. And the average lifespan of a woman was not eighty-six a thousand years ago. It was thirty-six." Therefore, most women weren't living long enough to achieve what we now commonly refer to as menopause.

As much of history has been penned by men, our framework for studying menstruation historically is kind of limited. A lot of what we know, or think we know, comes from pulling back the curtain on the proverbial Red Tent, which is not something lost to ancient history. The practice of sequestering women away to menstruate is still very much in practice all over the world. Menstrual huts are still prevalent in some parts of India, and attempts to ban these *gaokors*, as they're called, have been unsuccessful. The National Human Rights Coalition visited well over two hundred of them in 2015 and found that since they're public property, no one specific is responsible for their maintenance. Most of them lack a proper bed. They're also typically placed in fairly remote settings, and should a woman end up there alone for the duration (as is often the case), she's vulnerable to predators. This practice begins as soon as a young woman gets her first period, and therefore, 23 percent of girls in India drop out of school when they start menstruating.

Although the most obvious justification for hiding menstruating women away comes straight from the biblical "periods make you unclean" narrative, anthropologists and sociologists have also suggested that husbands can exact more control over their wives and daughters through enforcing their menstrual hut stay: they know exactly where they are, because they've disallowed them from being anywhere else for at least five days of the month.

The biblical passage most often cited is Leviticus 15:19. Depending on which translation you're reading, menstruation is referred to as "discharge," "regular flow of blood," "menstrual period," a woman's "impurity," or, in the King James—her "issue." The warning being that if anyone (read: a man) touched a woman during the week she was bleeding, he'd be unclean for the rest of the day. The specificity is interesting here: women certainly don't consistently bleed for seven days; it can be more or less by a rather large margin. And why would the person touching the woman only be made dirty "till the evening"? The Bible also notes, in nearby passages, that a woman who bears a male child is unclean for seven days after the birth, and that when she's on her period, everything she comes into contact with is also made filthy. Like some kind of Menstrual Midas Touch.

What's important to keep in mind here is that it wasn't really about the blood itself—no one's really worried about staining chairs. The problem is where the blood's coming from. I mean, if a gladiator shed his blood on your recently swept kitchen floor, you'd feel blessed. But, quite literally, God forbade a woman's menstrual effluent from touching you or anything you loved.

The problem with a woman's "blood" was really not the problem at all: vaginas were the problem. To extrapolate, women's sexuality was the problem. Women having agency of their bodies was the problem. And while these social mores were certainly explicit through other teachings, menstruation took on a symbolic quality for womanly wiles, for female evils, for the feminine mystique. The lore of a creature—whether witch or siren or selkie—who could bleed for a week and not die endures.

A researcher and academic named Sara Read shed some much-needed light on the menstrual practices of yore in her paper "'Thy Righteousness Is but a Menstrual Clout': Sanitary Practices and Prejudice in Early Modern England." Indeed, as she introduces her topic, she points out that there's no great wealth of information on the subject. First-person accounts by women throughout history are limited by a peculiar social paradox: menstruation is both mundane and wildly taboo.

Throughout history, men have told very specific tales about menstruation—either from the "informed" medical perspective or as a salacious literary device on the part of poets and philosophers. Read, in fact, cites several poems, one of which is "By All Love's Soft, Yet Mighty Powers," by John Wilmot, Earl of Rochester, which begins thusly:

> *By all love's soft, yet mighty powers,*
> *It is a thing unfit,*
> *That men should fuck in time of flowers,*
> *Or when the smock's beshit.*

Rochester's charming little ditty goes on to recount his experience of having sex with a prostitute, who he is disgusted to find is on her period (the "time of flowers"). Rochester goes on to elucidate that while he enjoys sex with prostitutes, what would really get him rock-hard would be if the woman would stop up her menstrual flow while they were doing it so his dick wouldn't get a nosebleed (in the poem he does actually make this exact comparison).

The boner-crushing qualities of menstruation hardly began with Rochester: Read also reminds us of the story of Hypatia, a Greek mathematician and astronomer in the fourth century, a woman who did not suffer fuckboys gladly.

As the legend goes, one of Hypatia's students became infatuated with her, his lust becoming all the more aggressive the more she rebuffed him. She, naturally, grew weary of his attempts to pressure her into having sex she didn't want to have, so she showed him her bloodied menstrual rags and told him he was a pig. The feminine mystique having been shattered, he was immediately and irreparably repulsed by her.

One could argue that the lad was equally repulsed by Hypatia's strength, and probably also humiliated by the fact that she had no interest in him whatsoever. What ultimately translated into culture from that event was that menstruation was a sure-fire way to cure lust. That's a bias that still exists today, despite the fact that we essentially accept menstruation as an inevitable, and therefore natural, part of life.

It's interesting that so many women have held onto the belief, or instinct even, that menstruation is natural, when history has dictated that to bleed is not just unnatural, but condemnable. One might wonder if viewing menstruation as natural is less about accepting biological purpose and more a matter of ownership. Of identity, even.

Whether one can learn to be at peace with her period on a personal level or not, menstruation still puts women at many practical disadvantages—some of which, over the past few decades, have proven life threatening.

An editorial published in the *British Journal of Sports Medicine* called out clinical researchers in a study on exercise that blatantly excluded women. The rationale for leaving them out? Because they get periods. "A review of 1,382 sport and exercise research studies involving over 6 million participants, from 2011 to 2013, found the representation of women to be 39%," wrote the authors. "The complexities of the menstrual cycle are considered major barriers to the inclusion of women in clinical trials."

This isn't really news to anyone, as the writers of this editorial continue to point out: historically, clinical trials (especially for those testing out new, yet-to-be-approved drugs) were done exclusively in men. Testing on women, it was argued, risked damaging an unborn fetus that she didn't know existed. Women were also perceived as being more "physiologically variable"—which is not necessarily untrue or even unfair. Men don't have a cyclical physiological experience akin to menstruation. One could argue (and they do in the rationales for these studies) that using only men would yield more consistent results. More consistent results mean the study is done faster and more accurately, which equals less money spent.

The exact reason that they exclude women (to save money) could potentially cost patients and health-care systems more money in the long run. Why? Because those physiological differences between men and women mean that there are probably differences in their responses to medications, treatment, and surgery. If we study men because they're easy and cheap to study, we're leaving out the realities of an entire patient population. A major study showing that aspirin reduced the risk of heart disease and stroke, for example, did not include women. In 1993, it was this study that prompted the ban on women participating in clinical trials to be lifted. That year, Congress passed the National Institutes of Health (NIH) Revitalization Act, mandating that NIH-funded research include women and minorities.

It probably comes as no surprise, then, that many of the drugs on the market in the 1980s were later withdrawn once people figured out that they didn't work as well in women, or, in some cases, caused serious side effects.

Methandrostenolone, for example, also known as Dianabol, a commonly used steroid, became notorious in the Olympic doping scandals—which was pretty much exactly what the physician who began prescribing it to Olympic athletes intended. He had suspected (correctly) that the Russians had been doping their athletes in the 1960s, so he started prescribing steroids to US athletes. The clinical trials for the steroid had been done, of course, in male athletes.

Dbol, as it was often affectionately called, was basically oral testosterone with a few extra carbon bonds to reduce estrogen conversion. It didn't actually work out that way, though; instead, it created a potent estrogen in the body. Those large "pecs" in bodybuilders were basically abnormally large breast tissue from excess estrogen, and the weight gain perceived from the steroid was really just water weight from bloating, also caused by the estrogen.

Those quick gains that are characteristic of steroids are, oddly enough, extremely familiar to most menstruating women. The water weight a woman gains before her period each month can be severe—ten pounds in a day—but it isn't permanent. The male Olympians using Dbol as a kick-starter for injectable steroid regimens were in for a rude awakening about its long-term side effects. When the drug came under fire for "off-label use," many of the athletes who were using it were women seeking to compete at a higher level. Since the drug hadn't been explicitly tested in women, the ill-effects of the drug, as reported by the female cohorts, probably helped get it off the market.

One would probably expect men and women to have different reactions to steroids, as the drug would be interacting with different existing base hormones. But researchers would later discover that

biological sex plays a role in the metabolism of lots of drugs. Everything from antidepressant response to anesthesia complications can
be influenced by the physiological differences between women and
men. Women, for one thing, have a higher ratio of fat to lean body
mass, which means that drugs relying on lipids may be metabolized
more quickly in a woman's body than in a man's. The implications
of such differences are vast—different dosages, for example, may be
necessary to achieve the same result.

Where a woman is in her menstrual cycle also influences how
her body metabolizes, well, anything. Researchers know this: that's
why, when they do include women in trials, they design the research
so that women will be participating early in their cycles, when their
hormones are most similar to a man's. Periods, then, have become
something of an exclusionary pathology.

Once my period became a pathology—once it became more of a
chronic condition than a monthly visitor, when the ramifications of
this so-called natural phenomenon gone rogue started to dictate my
every move—I realized that it had already altered me. It had shifted
my sense of self, of identity. Endometriosis began to ruin my life long
before I had a name for it.

—⊛—

SIX MONTHS AFTER I RETURNED to Maine, Rebecca—who said
she had missed me and consistently worried about me since I'd left
school—wanted to come up for the summer, partly to live with me,
but also just because she loved Maine. With her helping me out with
rent, it seemed doable, at least in the short term. Besides, Maine in
the summer was awash with jobs, if only seasonal ones, and I had to
find some way to make money— preferably sitting down.

I settled into a small apartment right after my twentieth birthday. It was tiny, like tiny-house tiny, and had one bed that was situ-
ated in a nook, surrounded by walls of bookshelves. The back porch
overlooked a nature preserve that was striking in its beauty and untouched serenity. Rebecca came up as soon as school ended, having
found a job in Portland, which was a couple hours' drive away. Having grown up outside of Hartford, she didn't balk at the commute, not
if it meant she could do something she really wanted to do. I found a

job in an art gallery. It allowed me to work sitting down, and it was quiet and not very demanding.

Summer in Maine is extremely gradual: you get a few weeks at the beginning where it might be eighty degrees during the day, but it dips down to forty or fifty degrees at night. Eventually, one day in mid-June you languidly realize that it's almost 9 p.m. and it's still light outside. Memories of the pink light in Estelle's backyard would find me from time to time as I looked out at the trees in my own backyard, listening to the cicadas sing. The summer meandered on and so did I until one day in early July, when my entire life changed again: I fell in love for the first time, and it was anything but gradual.

There was a coffee shop in town that I frequented during the off-season because it was quiet and had a warm, homey aesthetic. By the height of summer, I was working downtown right across the street, amid the throngs of tourists. The café became my sanctuary, even as it filled up with unfamiliar faces.

One morning I was there having brunch with my friend Julia, and she leaned over the table rather conspiratorially and informed me that the barista wanted to ask me out. I had no idea where she'd gotten this idea from. If he had been kind to me, it was surely only because he was hoping for a good tip, and I couldn't blame him. But beyond that—why would any man in his right mind make a pass at me? I was a hot mess. I looked as shitty as I felt most days. Not that I had ever been particularly good-looking. I never had been, and it had never bothered me all that much. I figured that being smart was enough for what I wanted out of life, and if that didn't entice a man, then, whatever, I'd live alone with half a dozen dogs and get to maintain my preference for sleeping with a fan year-round. Perfect!

When I took our plates up to the counter before we left, I suppose I made eyes at him. He asked where I went to school; even though I'd left, I told him Sarah Lawrence. I was still hoping that one day I'd go back, somehow. Besides, I *had* studied there, it wasn't exactly a lie.

A few days later, I showed up to work only to get a call from my boss saying that we weren't opening up for a few hours because her daughter was having a baby. She said, "Go get a cup of coffee, I'll call in a bit."

So I walked across the street to the café. There he was, smiling away, entertaining customers. I thought perhaps I had imagined it, but I could have sworn his eyes lit up when he saw me. He brought coffee to my table and some of it slopped onto my lap. He apologized profusely, but I brushed it off. As we sat there, I tried to sip my coffee the way a woman might like to be seen with a glass of wine— gracefully, and with a practiced air of judging whether or not she's had too much. I caught him staring at me and I smiled. When he asked me to dinner, I said yes.

Although I readily accepted the invitation, I was nervous about having to explain almost immediately that I couldn't really eat anything. It was either that or risk vomiting all over him mid-date, which might be highly arousing in some obscure mammalian courting rituals, but not with humans.

We went to a deli on the corner, a place that always made me salivate because it was full of things like onions and red peppers, which I hadn't eaten in years. I nibbled at a depressingly bland sandwich and got periodically lost in his big, sparkling blue eyes. Though we had only just met, and didn't even know any of the same people, we immediately felt a strange kinship. I was so comfortable around him that I joked that maybe we had known one another in a previous life. He told me my aura was purple. We laughed and exchanged numbers.

That weekend, I wrote in my journal, "Max—the boy—wants to take me sailing tomorrow." I found myself thinking of him, daydreaming, even: the certain air with which he entered a room, his gait quick but not hurried, directed but not premeditated. He had a dancer's sureness on his feet. His hands were nimble, finely tuned. Steady. I fell in love with him easily. Then I started to fall into this new kind of love with the entire world around me, which, for the first time since I'd gotten sick, seemed to be spinning madly on once again. I also hoped I might acquire a little self-love in the process—a process which I, of course, heavily romanticized. With his help, I wondered, would I learn to see the beauty in the soft rocking of my pelvis as I strode down the street? Or in the way my fingers wrapped themselves around a doorknob? What, I wondered, would it feel like to be regarded as unequivocally lovely? To be truly elegant? Would he find himself captivated by watching me sleepily pour coffee, yawning

unselfconsciously in his presence? Would he tremble pleasantly at the
sound of my throaty laugh, perceiving it as silvery echoes filling the
room and making him laugh, too?

Later that first week, I added to my journal: "Max took me sailing. He wants to date me. I know because of his hands. I'm terrified."

I was still a virgin at twenty. The last boyfriend I had had was
during my senior year of high school. The enduring memory I have
of him was the one night we spent together at his apartment. It was a
few weeks before I left for college: a grotesquely hot summer night,
which is usually the setting for these stories. We spoke in hushed
tones in his darkened living room, smoking American Spirits and
listening to music. Outside, in an act of nature's compassion, it began
to rain.

It was late, and I didn't want to drive on sweaty roads, so I let
him tuck me in on his couch. Not long after he went down the hall
to his bedroom, I followed, intending to linger desirably in his darkened doorway—when a familiar twist in my gut reminded me that I
was on my period. So, I stood semi-awkwardly in the doorway instead. A fan blew hopelessly in the corner of his too-small, sweltering
room. He cracked a window and put on some music—Explosions in
the Sky. I still remember it. "Your Hand in Mine" was the song. He
slung his arm around my waist and we listened to the storm outside. I
stayed awake long after he fell asleep, worrying that I'd bleed all over
his bed in the night. As I lay there, I was awash with the feeling of
being felt. When I woke up the next morning, he made me breakfast.
The tenderness of that memory is almost more revealing to me than
when I did eventually lose my virginity. The gift of human contact he
gave me was quintessential and irreplaceable.

I wasn't someone who had been regularly hugged or kissed as a
child. Physical affection of any kind, while I yearned for it, eluded
me. This had been one of those defects I'd identified about myself
years ago in therapy with Jane; I had certainly wanted to work on it,
but I just hadn't had that many opportunities. Sarah Lawrence hadn't
exactly been the epicenter of heat-seeking, hot-blooded, heterosexual
men—nor was the dance world.

Nor were the options in small-town Maine particularly bountiful. Even if they had been, given my state of ill-health, I had very

little faith that a summer flirtation would amount to anything, though Rebecca had warned me not to overthink it. Max and I had experienced an undeniable spark. I had never felt like that about another person before. I'd never experienced the pull of passionate physical attraction. We didn't even have to be close enough to touch: if he merely stepped into my orbit when we were walking down the street, or reached over to shift his car into gear and nearly grazed my thigh, my entire body became aglow.

One night, he picked me up for dinner and then took an unfamiliar turn on our way back. I asked where we were going, and he said, "I'm trying to maintain a modicum of surprise here." I snorted at his ten-point vocabulary word and fell a little bit more for him. He took me to one of his favorite places, a slant of rocky shoreline that overlooked the harbor. It was kind of hidden away, accessible by a beaten dirt path through the woods, and was, I admit, rather romantic.

He opened his arms to me, so that I could settle against his chest to watch the sun set. The minute I sank back into his arms, I was plagued with a feeling of emptiness. I couldn't feel his arms, I could only feel myself. After a few very long moments spent like this, he sighed.

"If I let myself, I'm going to fall madly in love with you," he said. "But I'm afraid that you won't be able to love me back."

I turned my face to look up at him, completely breathless. "The only thing I'm sure of," he continued, "is that if I let myself fall in love with you, I will never love anyone as intensely again."

For once in my life I was speechless. Fighting the urge to come up with something equally amorous to say, I willed myself to be in that moment, to live in it, to *feel* it. When I got home that night, I wrote down every single second of it in my journal, recognizing, I suppose, that something quite serious had happened to me.

The following evening, Rebecca was out for the night working, so Max came over. We talked for hours without running out of things to say. Talking led to kissing, which I was extremely bad at and I knew it. He was patient. He tried to provide some guidance, though he did find it amusing that I seemed to be able to only kiss with my head tilted one way. I assured him that I was very good at taking direction and a quick study. I was a dancer who was, admittedly, not as good at improvisation as some. But if you gave me the choreography and an idea of what the dance was meant to convey, I could pick it up. This made sense to him, but he explained—a bit to my dismay—that what made kissing fun was the unexpected.

"Don't do back exactly what I'm doing. Change it up a little," he said, settling back against my bed. Great, I thought. It's improv. He noticed my hesitation and thought for a minute, then tried a different tack, using a language in which we'd already established our mutual fluency.

In the end it was his more technical illustration—a slightly clunky analogy using thermodynamic stability—that, surprisingly, helped.

Then, somewhat inexplicably, *geekily* aroused, I joined him on the bed. My shirt came off first, and I had not been wearing a bra—a decision which, as a then-single woman with chronic pain in the middle of July, I don't have to justify to anyone. It did seem like altogether too quick a reveal to me, but he wasn't disappointed. I blushed severely, a full-bodied rosiness that may have been warm and lovely, but also panic-inducing. No one had ever seen my breasts before, let alone touched them this way. I wasn't yet accustomed to interpreting the type of unspoken communication that occurs in these situations, and I briefly considered asking for some kind of verbal reassurance, but I couldn't figure out how. I rightly assumed that something like, "Are they breasty enough?" would have ruined the magic. Instead, I tried to commit to the immersion learning experience.

Max's lips discovered the shoreline of my collarbones, his hot skin warming my face. His hands found my abdomen, his fingers climbing the lattice of my ribs, then slipping down to my lower pelvis with its slow healing scars. He was gentle, but moved with what I now understand was practiced finesse. He knew where he was going even if I didn't, and while I had a passing feeling of disappointment in myself for not knowing everything, I also recognized that it was an important exercise in trust. And a gentler side of me pointed out, of course, that there was a first time for everything. And some firsts were big, and the only one you got.

I had expected that if he put anything inside me—finger, phallus, what-have-you, it would hurt. Not necessarily because I had pain there to begin with, or because of all the painful pelvic exams in my life. I'd just grown up, like many young women do, being warned that "the first time hurts."

⁓⚶⊕

I OFTEN WONDER IF MY early sexual education may have, in a way, set me up for this fate. I was in the fifth grade, and there were two teachers: both female and in their late fifties. One of them was gregarious and open, and framed the conversation with multiple exclamation points: exciting!!! The other was gravely serious, probably a little repressed, and thoroughly mortified.

Take a wild guess as to who ended up teaching the girls.

While the laughter of the boys echoed from the classroom next door, the lot of us poor prepubescent females sat squirming in our seats as our long-faced teacher struggled to even utter the word "vagina." Hillary and I sat trying to reconcile what we thought we heard as "Velveeta," and I became increasingly frustrated that the boys were having a grand old time with their sex ed, and all I was feeling was embarrassed and guilty about something I didn't even understand—an emerging theme in my life.

At recess, we congregated on the playground's grassy knoll, forgoing our usual co-ed kickball game to debrief on our Very Important Lesson. While the boys alternately squealed and threw themselves head-first down the hill as they echoed their teacher's decree of "Sex is greeeeeat!," we girls sat at the top of the hill compulsively plucking blades of grass by the fistful. The boys ran around with their newly minted swagger, their sexual enlightenment, their permission for pleasure, and we blushed at the realization that, while we supposedly had been gifted with invaluable information regarding the mechanics, we hadn't been told a thing about how sex should feel, or why anyone would want to do it. Aside from the obvious: having a baby.

The boys, in short, had emerged from their side of the classroom double doors equipped with almighty knowledge to which the girls were not privy. Now, with Max, I once again found myself in a situation where men somehow knew more about what was happening inside of my body than I did. But this time, I was quite literally positioned to discover, and perhaps claim, my sexual power. I was electrified. Even the tickling sensation on my back from my own hair—which I had let grow long, too lazy to cut it—was a full-body awakening.

Max and I didn't have intercourse that night, but the sexual exploration we did undertake hurt—and deeply. Starting in my pelvis and rising up into my chest, everything ached for days afterward, and I accepted this as normal. No one had ever prepared me for anything different, so I wasn't terribly worried about it. And, pain aside, it had all been rather dramatic and interesting. I felt rather dramatic and interesting myself.

The next morning, after he left, I rolled over to face the empty bed, and my blood-stained sheets, and the throbbing pain, and the lingering scent of him on my pillow, and suddenly I was spooked. Had I done something bad? Was it supposed to hurt that much? What did it mean that he had touched me that way, that he'd slept in my bed, our limbs tangling in the night? I rolled over and stared at the ceiling for a long time, wishing I had someone to talk to about it.

More than that, I felt that I had experienced a little magic. I suppose I wanted someone to tell me it was okay.

Later that week, when I had my session with Jane, I told her the story from start to finish, practically on a single breath. I felt like I was in confession, and somehow telling someone these things, even though she wasn't saying anything, made it real.

I looked up at her, catching my breath, and then, I started to cry. "I don't know what's happening," I said, laughing through my tears.

"This is falling in love," she said knowingly. "It's a gift—not him, but you. You're going to learn so much about yourself."

"And it's okay?" I asked meekly, reaching up to wipe my eyes.

"Yes, it's okay," she tutted, a bemused glint in her eye. "It's wonderful."

I studied her face for a moment—something I rarely did. It was my tendency not to look at her very often, if at all, during our hour-long sessions. She had, years before, told me in a therapeutically relevant manner that she had been widowed fairly young. Her grief had been carefully compartmentalized, much to her credit, but it still glistened behind her eyes like an eternal flame. To realize, in that moment, the depth of her grief also required me to acknowledge the depth of the love she'd known. I wondered if I was on the precipice of knowing that kind of love myself.

Our session was over, so I stood to leave. She stood, too.

"I'm so happy for you," she said. At first, I thought she meant she was glad to see me having a semi-age-appropriate experience for once in my life. And maybe she did mean that. But I also think she meant that she was happy, maybe even a little bit proud, that I had been brave.

I smiled, tears still blurring my vision.

Then, overcome by a strange joy, I hugged her.

⸻🕮⸻

A FEW WEEKS AFTER MAX and I started dating, I came down with a horrible case of strep throat. This was a fate that has befallen me with alarming consistency my whole life. I probably should have had my tonsils out, if they still do that. Even when I was little, one bout of strep would make my tonsils swell up for months, giving me the voice of a beleaguered, grisly old woman who smoked a pack a day. This particular bout was no different.

I fell ill over the weekend and knew I'd need to go to the emergency room for a throat culture and some antibiotics. I'd had strep so many times in my life that all it took was a specific feeling in my left ear canal, and I knew I was headed for the full-blown thing. I never have minded being a patient when it's something like strep. Doctors like it when the problem is easy to diagnose and fairly uncomplicated to fix—and who can blame them? They'd do a throat swab. It would be positive for strep. I'd get antibiotics. I'd push fluids. I'd get better. Max was working, and I had quickly become too feverish to safely drive, so his father offered to take me.

I'd only just met Max's parents, Simon and Maggie. The four of us had gone to dinner and played Scrabble. I would later learn that I'd won them over by playing the word "trove."

Simon was a quiet, rather serious man with excellent taste in hats. When he asked me questions, I felt a bit like I was at a job interview. That actually worked well in my favor, as I'd always been more confident in those types of professional situations than in the improvisation of casual discourse. And I loathe small talk.

Maggie was older than I'd expected. My mother had had me young and still hadn't hit menopause—Maggie, then, was closer in age to my grandmother. We had immediate common ground, though, as she had been a dancer in her youth, and it showed. She was quite fetching: lithe, graceful, and almost disarmingly kind and conversationally affable.

Simon was a bit more restrained, though not altogether humorless. So, on the day he accompanied me to the hospital for a strep test, I was a bit taken aback when he offered to let me crash on their couch until Max got out of work. I was too exhausted to politely protest, and as I fell into a fever-stupor on their couch, he put on a kettle and offered a piece of satisfied wisdom from their sunny kitchen:"You're in the right place. Just be sick. You don't have any other responsibility."

I must have felt at least a little bit safe, because I fell into a deep, febrile sleep. I was roused from it an indeterminate number of hours later, when the house around me had grown dark. Maggie was gently nudging me, a thermometer in her hand.

"Sorry to wake you sweetie, but I'm worried," she said, and she did sound worried, which I found almost comical, because I was so unaccustomed to being fussed over. She brushed her cool palm against my forehead and stuck the thermometer in my mouth, then proceeded to ask me if I'd rather sleep upstairs, in Max's bed or their guest bed. I moaned. I could hardly keep my eyes open, and I was afraid that if I tried to move, I'd fall right onto the floor. The couch was actually pretty cozy—and I'd slept on enough couches in my day to know.

"You can stay right here, as long as you're comfortable," Maggie replied, which meant that my non-answer had conveyed the right sentiment. The thermometer beeped and she took it out of my mouth as she asked, "Do you want something to eat? Or some tea maybe?"

"I might take some tea later," I croaked, my fear of being impolite finally overcoming the shards of glass in my throat. "Thank you."

As I drifted back to sleep, listening to his parents tutting away nervously in the kitchen, hearing the screen door smack as Max came in, feeling him lift me from the couch a moment or so later, I

remembered what he'd said to me in the car on that night he'd introduced me to them: "They'll love you. They'll make you a part of this
family. You have to be ready for that."

I wasn't. And like everyone else who had tried to love the darkness out of me—neither were they.

SHORTLY THEREAFTER, I LOST MY virginity to Max in a sunny corner bedroom on borrowed sheets with a higher thread count than I
felt I deserved. Not in the least because I knew that eventually, if not
at that particular moment of penetration, I would bleed on them.

I had been instructed throughout my life—by older women, by
books, by society—that I wouldn't enjoy my first time, but that gradually sex would get better, so I should just stick it out. It was true that
the first time was painful, but because I had been anticipating that, I
wasn't particularly surprised or disappointed. What did surprise me
was that, despite the pain of penetration, I really liked everything
else sex involved, the vast majority of which was brand new to me.

For one thing, I had a great deal to learn about penises: I was at
first rather embarrassed by the fact that I had seen precious few of
them in my life before the opportunity arose to put one inside of me.
I had not watched the requisite porn as a teenager (which would have
been an especially difficult feat to manage when I was sleeping on
people's living-room couches), and therefore I found the need to ask
a lot of questions. It's always been my nature to be fascinated, and it
seemed reasonable that my sexual awakening would present as good
a time to be astonished as any.

Max was patient with me. He'd "been with other women," as he
put it—something that seemed impressively classy coming from a
twenty-year-old—and I suppose he figured he'd seen enough vaginas
to have seen them all. Not that I asked: I was too enthralled by the
concept of a scrotum.

He subtly took the lead when penetration became imminent. I
don't know exactly how this was decided, but I'm sure it involved
some kind of definitive, practical statement from me. Something to
the tune of, "AFFIRMATIVE: I'm sufficiently lubricated and aroused
for this consensual sexual activity. PROCEED."

I remember thinking it felt like having your hand slammed in a car door. The pain was a deep ache, like a dull pinch, that resonated in my pelvis. My belly clenched, and I guess I made some God-awful noise, because he immediately looked down at me, a heaving breath away from a stilted apology.

I swallowed hard, tears pooling in the corners of my eyes and sliding down my cheeks as I smiled, telling him I was fine, to keep going. I had expected it to hurt, and it had hurt.

The problem was, it never stopped hurting—but it took me at least the first year of our relationship to admit that it was painful, that something was wrong.

At the end of that summer, Max and I moved in together. By then, I'd explained my situation, and although I wasn't going back to Sarah Lawrence, I was determined to do *something* with myself during the fall semester when Max went back to school. I had some money saved up, and so long as he was enrolled in school, his parents were helping him some. I tried to take a few classes at one of the other universities in the college town where we lived. I had also tried to start taking dance classes again. But my health continued to decline, and neither of those things, despite my best efforts, worked out beyond the first semester. Incidentally, Max ended up hating the program he was in. We were happy with each other but not with what we were doing, so we moved back to the town where we'd met, where his family was, so that he could figure out what he wanted to do next. I was left to figure out what I *could* do next.

Despite the pain that I continued to experience with intercourse, I fell in love with the intimacy of it. I had never spent so much time being physically close to another person. In our new little apartment, we slept in an overpriced queen-sized bed (our first joint purchase), and he was an incredible space heater at night. I loved sliding my feet between his calves to warm them up (which he didn't appreciate, I'm sure, but he'd still roll over and embrace me in his sleep). If I woke suddenly, some forgotten terror clawing at my guts, I would immediately calm upon realizing he had his arms around me, that I was safe.

On Christmases, we went to upstate New York with his family, and they were the best Christmases of my life. We'd sleep on a teeny tiny air mattress in a spare bedroom, and Maggie would pop her head

in to wake us up on Christmas morning. One year, when we sleepily stumbled out for breakfast, she remarked that when she'd opened
the door, we'd been asleep with our faces about a centimeter away
from each other, and she didn't know how we could possibly sleep
like that. But then she and Simon exchanged something of a knowing
glance. They sighed in unison, as though they had both remembered,
for a split second, what it felt like to be in love for the first time. Maggie did know—she'd just forgotten.

Years later, after Max and I broke up and I kept the apartment, I
would examine the bedroom in the early morning hours, contemplat-
ing the loss. For a long time afterward, the air in the room felt stale
and I kept it dark, the shadows of the creases in the sheets where we
had once lain intertwined, staying in crumpled stillness. I liked the
boneyard quality of the room—it suggested perpetuation. When I finally couldn't stand the scent of him hovering anymore, I opened the
windows, even though it was the dead of winter. I could practically
see my breath in front of me, and the sheets were icy against my skin.
When spring came, the room and I thawed, sunlight penetrating the
window and cutting diagonally across the bed, making it appear as
though it had been split right down the middle. It hadn't felt that way.

I had never experienced the freedom of physical touch before
Max—sexual or otherwise. And I only realized after he was gone
that it was the nonsexual intimacy, the nonsexual physical touch, that
was ultimately the most healing. The sexual element, though, gave
me a vital education of my body that would prove to be invaluable
later on. The knowledge that intercourse was intolerable because of
disease became an answer to a question I hadn't found a way to ask.

As the years passed and my illness only got worse, my body
seeming to be continuously giving up the fight, it wore on both Max
and me. We were only kids. Kids who had fallen into passionate love
for the first time. It was, in its way, absolute magic. But most magic
is about sleights of hand and misdirection. Ours, in the end, was no
different.

Max had brought with him a family: two parents who were perhaps a little overprotective, but fundamentally good, and willing, and
loving. No family is without its darkness, and mistakes, and loathing.
But when there's support, and affirmation, and love, to balance the

suffering out a little, you manage. In retrospect, I think my relationship to Max's parents—which was at times more complicated and
emotionally wrought than my relationship with their son—provided
the most lasting lessons.

The first year we were together, we went to Simon and Maggie's
for the week of Thanksgiving. On one of those evenings, he went off
to visit some of his friends, and I stayed behind, because I didn't feel
well. I don't think he was too disappointed—we both understood that
we needed time to be with our friends separate from one another, and
I wasn't going to harp on him about where he was, or what he was
doing, or who he was with. First, because I trusted him. But second,
because I had a lot of other stuff on my mind and didn't want the responsibility of "mothering" him.

I'd recently acquired all of my medical records—in part because
I was trying to be certain that the piles of medical bills I had were
all accurate—and in the process, I began to reopen the emotional
wound of leaving Sarah Lawrence. This particular night, I was in the
living room at his parents' house, chatting absently with Maggie after
dinner. She innocently inquired about my health, not realizing the
Pandora's Box she'd opened.

Despite the fact that I hadn't known her that long, something let
go inside of me. I told her the whole gruesome story—more than
I'd told Max at that point. To my horror, as I flipped through page
after page after page of medical records, I started to heave with
tears. Immediately embarrassed, I tried to gather myself—and my
paperwork—so that I could retreat upstairs. I didn't want to make her
uncomfortable. I also wasn't quite ready for Max, let alone his whole
family, to know what a goddamn nightmare I really was.

She rose from her chair and I felt a pang of hurt and shame,
thinking she was getting up to leave because of my display of emotion. Instead, she came over to the couch and wrapped me up in a
hug. At first I didn't know what to do. I hadn't been hugged very
much, certainly never held, during the years of my young life where
most people learn how to give and receive physical affection. If I experienced physical affection at all, it was a brief "there, there" type
of hug, where the other person would rapidly pat my back to signal
that we'd touched for long enough and it was time to disengage. That

wasn't what Maggie was offering, though. She had fully embraced me such that my head was beneath her chin, my tears staining her very nice, sweet-smelling sweater.

She didn't say a word. She didn't chide me or dismiss me with a "Now that's quite enough of that," pat-pat-pat on the shoulder. She let me cry until my whole body was numb. Other than the sound of my own sniffling, the room fell into such a hush that I could hear her heart beating against my ear. Though fear and anguish had risen up in me, there was something incredibly tranquil in that moment. I calmed, and expected the "there, there" dismissal to be issued, but she only waited. When my tears cycled up again, she held on as though it were the most obvious response. As though it were the only response. As though it were something that humans knew, instinctively, to do.

At some point, a more ancient grief welled up and began to flood me. A deeply buried, nascent part of me could have stayed on that couch for eternity, and was petrified by the prospect of being released back into the wild.

But the more mature, cerebral—and at times, callous—part of me resented that I'd even let it happen. That I had let my emotions overcome me when my ability to compartmentalize had long been my most remunerative asset. I was alternatively humiliated by the enormity of my need for comfort and heartsick thinking about how little of it I had experienced in my young life. At least in the way that Max's mother was providing it.

That all being said, it felt nice when Max held me, too. I felt small and somewhat effeminately delicate in his strong caveman arms. My evolutionary instincts were satisfied that he could build me a hut, if required. For this very primal reason, being held by Max—or any man—felt very distinct from the more gestational embrace of a woman.

With Max, being held was pleasant but not exactly calming. It felt good to be close to him because I was attracted to him and aroused by him. Having his arms around me, in other words, was a nice feeling, but one that invariably led to, "Okay, now let me suck your dick." It was the "hurts so good" intensity of attraction. His embrace was molecularly energizing.

I've had strange moments throughout my life where it feels as though I am expanding infinitely out into the universe, as though every double helix of my DNA were unfurling. It felt like every atom of my body was being drawn back to the cosmos by some unseen force, and was trying to return to whatever star I came from. In these moments, I find myself desperately wanting to be held. But more than held—stilled.

Physical closeness with a man (sometimes as little as proximity—touching isn't strictly necessary) inspires sexual stirrings in me because I'm straight. At least that's what I assume. I've never been stirred in that sexual way by physical closeness to a woman. Inspired to sob uncontrollably for no discernible reason, yes, but not sexually aroused. Not that I would have minded if I had been, of course, they've just always felt like two distinct phenomena to me.

In my situation, being straight has probably simplified the process of parsing unmet emotional yearnings from other instigators of intimacy. If I'd been physically yearning for women—emotionally and sexually—I think it would have been incredibly challenging to examine and isolate the various threads of meaning within those experiences. Certainly there have been women in my life who have interpreted the mighty need I have for their affection to be sexual. I suspect because they have never felt the touch-hunger of a mother-starved child. The women I've met who have known that yearning immediately know what I'm talking about, and they, too, regard it as being fundamentally different, and separate from, their sexuality. I doubt it even exists on the same plane of consciousness as sexual desire. Freud would disagree—but who asked him?

This separateness is evidenced by two important points: first, although I am not always aware of my mother-yearning in the moment—only realizing in retrospect that I was inexplicably, emotionally upset by the presence of a woman—I am always aware of my sexuality when I'm engaged with a man. True, sometimes when a man is trying to flirt with me, I don't realize it. But that has more to do with my self-esteem than my perceptive abilities. Sexual attraction is glaringly obvious and easy to understand in the face of a more subtle, pernicious, and at times smothering need for the love of a parent.

Humans have, for millennia, pursued the arc of falling in love and being sexual creatures. Even when we get burned by love, we keep on looking for a match. We strike until we hit a spark; we move through space seeking that blissful friction of attraction. We rally for it, we race straight into it and leap, we dive, we plunge into love because even when it hurts, it's good. And when it's good? Oh, it is so truly, madly, deeply good.

The exhaustive quest for mother-love is nothing like that. It never feels good. We can understand why people want to fall in love again, why a sexual craving is enough to splinter the mind from its conscience. We're biologically hardwired to find a mate, but we're not born prepared to spend our lives yearning for a mother. We're supposed to be born and nurtured throughout our young lives so that we can live long enough to fulfill our sociobiological prophecy to fornicate, propagate, and spoil *The Walking Dead* for our coworkers.

There is no wiring, no sympathetic nervous system or empathetic external system that exists to help us out beyond the initial survival of maternal neglect. Technically, evolution dictates that if the baby doesn't bond to the mother or caregiver, it dies. It's actually extremely cut-and-dried, there's no subtlety here. It's beyond being fed and given a place to sleep. Do I really need to bring up Harry Harlow's monkeys again? Because I will.

LATER, WHEN EVERYTHING BEGAN TO unravel, the prospect of losing Max became greater than losing the man I loved. It was losing an entire family that loved me.

In the face of uncertainty, of true challenges and disappointing realities, love is sometimes not enough. The years I spent with Max were largely happy ones. We traveled together, went sailing, were often stopped on the street by complete strangers who said seeing two people so in love had brightened their day. And we were in love. But it wasn't enough. I wasn't enough.

I came to understand that sex would always hurt for me, and that therefore I probably wouldn't be having much of it. While this never seemed to get a rise out of any doctor when I fretted over it, once I

started taking Max with me to appointments, and he corroborated—
or better yet, expressed his own frustration—suddenly it seemed
like doctors started to listen. I was extremely peeved to have made
this observation. It either meant that they hadn't believed me in the
absence of Max as an alibi, or that they had believed me, but my
suffering alone wasn't enough to inspire action. Becoming a disappointment to a man, though, seemed to do the trick.

Max in tow, I went back to Dr. Paulson. Now that they knew I
couldn't put out like a woman should, they seemed to have an abundance of suggestions. I tried birth control. I got an IUD. I did pel-
vic-floor physical therapy until it became too excruciating to continue.
I have, in the name of pain management, had a varied assortment of
objects inserted into my vagina: hands, garlic cloves, polished stone,
colorful plastic "expanders" that are actually just medical-grade dil-
dos, slick transducers and icy speculums, catheters, swabs, scalpels,
and gauze. I saw homeopaths and naturopaths and took all kinds of
tinctures and pill-pods. I drank raspberry tea until I could no longer
stand the smell of it. I tried castor oil packs, I tried TENs units (that
is, transcutaneous electrical nerve stimulation), and I held electric
heating pads against my bare skin until they burned me. I lived in,
and for, hot bathwater.

The gynecologists told us to try different positions, angles, and
speeds, though I'd insisted that we'd already done that and would
have thought that was obvious. We were a pair of virile twenty-
somethings, so how did they not assume we had already repurposed
every surface of our home and several undisclosed public locales
for the express purpose of our mutual sexual gratification? I'd been
sneaking peeks at *Cosmopolitan* since at least the age of thirteen,
and Max had no doubt been a connoisseur of Internet pornography
for years, since all '90s kids learned the hard way that White House
Dot Com would not help us with our history reports.

Beyond that, I was dubious that sexual positions with names like
"The Viennese Oyster" or "Alligator Fuckhouse" were going to solve
the issue of painful sex. The latter sounded more likely to cause it.

Was I lubricated enough? They'd always ask this. I couldn't have
been more lubricated. But I wasn't sure how to prove that to them. I

have to say, of all the issues I've had gynecologically, wetness has never been one of them. I wish I could be proud of that fact, but it's proven a major impediment. It only stood to obfuscate the pain I experienced and somehow invalidated my claims of discomfort.

When it came to the pain, I had a difficult time articulating that it wasn't at the opening of my vagina, which was what doctors usually thought when I said "sex hurts." Vaginismus is very real: it's a condition where the vaginal wall and opening contract involuntarily to prevent penetration. Despite the fact that anecdotal evidence suggests it's fairly common, it has not been well studied. This was not where or why sex hurt for me—at least not when it started. Over time, my body did attempt, however, to involuntarily guard against the pain it came to expect—pain that would resound in my pelvis during coitus—and eventually that meant I stopped getting to the point of penetrative sex at all.

The pain emanating from my pelvis was much deeper than the pain women get with vaginismus; it came from somewhere that seemed to me to be so deep as to be untouchable. It was heavy, full, aching. There was almost a soreness to it, like a tender bruise, but on the inside. The rhythm of penetration made what had become a constant, dull pain every day into a momentary swell of intense, staggering, asphyxiating pain. I buried my face in the pillow and waited for sex to feel like something I'd risk my life for. At first, I swallowed down the yelps, gritting my teeth against the sensation of my organs being ripped away from the pelvic wall, or torn up like plants by the stalk. Roots that I had put down with Max. Though I had been afraid at first, I had come to feel secured by them. Roots might trap and entangle, but they're nice sometimes: when you're grounded, not every gust of wind breaks your neck. Roots are also necessary for nourishment. For growth. So I braced myself against the pain of intercourse and told myself that growing hurt.

Afterward, when I would go to the bathroom to wash up and there would be blood, and undulating waves of nausea, and an ache that spread down into my upper thighs, I told myself that this was just how sex was. It didn't take very long for me to begin to dread sex altogether, despite the fact that I was madly in love with Max, very attracted to him, and certainly felt that I wanted to have sex with him. Over time, the anticipation of the pain made me reluctant. Max couldn't help but take the rejection personally. How could he not? I was turning away from him. I was wincing at his touch.

LESS THAN A MONTH AFTER Max and I moved back to the town where we'd first met, I got a job at a hospital. I was already familiar with its emergency room because of my own visits to it since leaving New York. There had been an opening in the medical records department, and the head of it took a chance and hired me. I am forever grateful to her for seeing something in a plucky, if not sickly, twenty-two-year-old girl with no college degree.

People are often surprised to hear that I still worked, as sick as I was, but the simple truth was that I didn't have a choice. I was in no position to be taken care of. What money I'd squirreled away had long run out, and the mounting medical debt was crushing. I couldn't afford to be sick. I didn't have the luxury of just healing.

The fact that I got a job didn't exactly lend any credibility to my assertions that I felt wretchedly ill. But beyond the simple fact that I had to earn money, I was desperate for my life to have something in it besides illness. It's worth noting that the job I undertook didn't ask much of me: I sat at a desk most of the day, had reasonable hours, plus paid vacation and sick days, and it was an elevator ride to the ER if things got particularly bad. I also did little else aside from work; there was no energy left for anything else, including things like cleaning house, having a social life, or putting effort into the relationship I was in—which I wanted to be in. I was just so tired that sleep was usually more attractive than anything else.

Sometimes, well-meaning people point out to me that if I hadn't *had* to work, if someone had taken care of me, if I could have properly recuperated the first time around, without having to worry about where I was going to live or pay my bills, maybe I wouldn't have gotten so sick. I suppose that may be true, but it's a slippery slope I'd rather not go down, because you could apply that logic to my entire life.

Once, years ago, during a particularly harrowing session with Jane, she had studied me from across the room, from the sanctity of her wingback chair. "Imagine if we could have plucked you out of there, given you to a different family," she mused. "With that mind of yours . . ." The rest of her thought hung suspended between us, and I hadn't dared reach for it.

My mind was about all I had left, so when I noticed that the hospital housed a small medical library, I took up residence whenever I could, purloining copies of journals to take back to my regular desk. Having access to medical journals would prove invaluable to me over the course of the next year. If my life was to be one of pain, I wanted to learn the best I could how to cope. More than that, I wanted to understand categorically what was causing it. Whatever it was, I wanted to be an expert in it.

That had more or less been my modus operandi as a kid: when my brother was diagnosed with autism, I wanted to learn everything about autism. When I figured out my mother had bulimia, I wanted to know everything about bulimia. In the face of scary things, knowledge was always a comfort to me. No matter what the subject was, if I could find a book or two about it, I could squash any anxiety that it might provoke. As my heroine Scully once said, "The answers are there, you just have to know where to look."

Sitting at my desk going through back issues of the *New England Journal of Medicine*, I thought I knew where to look, but I didn't find much about endometriosis. I understood what an ovarian cyst was, and why it happened, but endometriosis had always been only a partial answer in the back of my mind. Maybe it was a big deal, or maybe it wasn't. What little I found about it in semi-outdated textbooks of gynecology wasn't exactly informative.

So I began to broaden my search. Day after day, I saw history and physicals—neatly transcribed in medical records—shuffle across my desk. I heard doctors murmuring in the dictation room, saying words like "hyperlipidemia" and "angioederma," but they floated through the office devoid of context. Medical terminology came easily to me, though. If I was processing a chart or sending off a surgical note and encountered a term I didn't know, I'd write it down and spend my break trying to solve the puzzle of its origin. Learning the language of medicine truly is like learning another language altogether: the prefixes and suffixes, the Latin roots. Like any other language, it has its aphorisms, its slang, and its inside jokes.

It occurred to me that even though I was no longer in college, no longer getting an education in the proper way, I was still learning. Probably more than I would have on any ivy-coated campus, really, because my motivation was beyond a degree at this point. I was trying to save my life.

One of the first things I did was write up a very thorough History and Physical of myself—as though I were the doctor for a moment and not the patient. I typed it up neatly, using the same template any doctor would have, and threaded in all the proper terminology. Or what I knew of it, at least.

HX OF PRESENT ILLNESS:

Patient is a 22-year-old gravida 0 para 0 female who complains of persistent RLQ pain that began in the fall of 2010. Pt reports cyclic pelvic pain, heavy menstrual periods, chronic nausea, progressively worsening fatigue and muscle weakness. She has also had frequent bouts of swollen cervical and supraclavicular lymph nodes, which may not be clinically relevant. She reports RIGHT-sided abdominal pain, which she indicates is at McBurney's Point, that is worsened by activity and sexual intercourse and not relieved with rest. Previous imaging studies did not reveal any indication of appendicitis.

PAST MEDICAL HISTORY:
- RIGHT-sided lipoma in lower back, not believed to be clinically significant
- DX LAP 2010—endometriosis of the posterior cul-de-sac and LEFT paratubal ovarian cyst, aspirated and wrapped with Interceed. Torsion of LEFT fallopian tube
- Significant unintended weight loss > 30 lbs
- Hx of depression, anxiety, currently on Zoloft and in psychotherapy
- Chronic nausea, early satiety
- Chronic pelvic pain
- Pelvic peritoneal endometriosis
- Dyspareunia

One of the first questions I started asking was why I had such a specific and constant pain at McBurney's point—the palpable location of the appendix—if imaging had shown no appendicitis. Granted, medical imaging was not perfect: after all, back when I'd had that cyst—the one that twisted my fallopian tube all about—they hadn't seen hide nor hair of it on an ultrasound or CT scan. Besides, how could someone possibly have appendicitis for *two years*?

I figured I should start with what I already knew was in there, which was endometriosis. The next logical question was, could endometriosis slather itself all over your appendix and cause trouble? Although there wasn't a lot to read about endometriosis in the academic literature I had access to, there were a few studies that seemed to back this theory up. Certainly locations that were near reproductive organs—which are many, probably more than most women realize—could be vulnerable to lesions. Or could I have lesions on my intestines?

The appendix hypothesis was a rather nerve-wracking thought: If my appendix was covered in endometrial tissue, would I eventually develop a more acute case of appendicitis? Or would it just simmer on and on, slowly leaching infection into my body? In either case, I'd need to do something about it. Or rather, convince someone with a scalpel and a license to practice medicine to do something about it. And would removing my appendix even solve the problem? Maybe if it was removed, the tissue would just come back, filling up the space where it had been.

Once I got a proper handle on the medical library, I had access to more databases and academic journals than I've ever had since—the benefit of health-care-system employment that surpasses even affiliation with an academic institution. I started looking for phrases like "chronic appendicitis" or "smoldering appendicitis" in my search for clinical evidence. What I found initially was that most medical professionals didn't believe it was possible for an appendix to be chronically inflamed. An appendix could get cancer, sure—that's what killed Audrey Hepburn—but the term "chronic appendicitis" was limited and hotly debated. The idea of subacute appendicitis, though, led me a little further down a path toward an answer.

Appendicitis seems common because it's a fairly regular pop-culture trope: if you need a sudden, nonfatal, but disruptive medical event to befall a character, appendicitis is a good option. It can start and be resolved over the course of a single twenty-minute episode.

Recall that your appendix is that little worm-like organ that hangs off the end of your large intestine, the part called your *cecum*. When an appendix becomes inflamed, the pain tends to start around the belly button. Then it progresses down toward the right hip bone (though not always) and lingers about midway, at McBurney's point. As you might expect, like many terms in medicine, this one is eponymous. Charles McBurney wrote about palpating this area as a diagnostic tool for appendicitis. However, medical historians don't seem to agree on whether or not he was the first to identify it—or just the first to write about it.

In any case, I thought about McBurney's point a lot—because it was exactly where I had this very particular, unrelenting pain. I certainly had pain in other areas of my pelvis and my lower back, but it was more diffuse. In this one spot, however, even back in the emergency room in New York years before, I had insisted there *was* something. Sometimes it felt like a heavy, hot stone. Other times it was like a balloon that was near-bursting—particularly when I walked at a good clip or attempted to run. I assume that, had I not already been forced to give up dance, any twisting or torquing of my body would have been equally offensive.

Even a light jostling—like going over a bump in the car—made it flare up momentarily. I'd often press my hand against the spot, a breath of air hissing through my teeth as I waited for it to calm again.

Intercourse was becoming intolerable for the same reason. Not only did it cause a deep, radiating ache in my pelvis and lower back, but each thrust felt as though it was jabbing whatever thing was inside of me. The pains, while distinct from one another, were in a sort of dance—a searing duet. Sometimes they happened all at once, a cacophony of heat and pressure and dull aches that I couldn't seem to parse out. Like there was a tangled ball of string pulsing in my core, and I couldn't peel away each individual string. I couldn't untie it. Then, other times, one would fade away into the background, like a hum. A shadow of something more demanding, more attention seeking. It would whisper in the shadows somewhere behind a bone while the other stepped forward, grabbing my ribs and yanking down. Grabbing my guts and twisting. And in those moments I could tell you where the pain was, I could point and press—but I couldn't tell you what it was. I gleaned little helpful information from anatomical drawings and three-dimensional plastic models. What I wanted to do was slice open my belly and have a little look-see.

And then, one day, an opportunity presented itself as I was wheeling my jingly little metal cart through the hospital corridors. You know, like a shopping cart with a rickety wheel? I had a little metal cart like that, and I'd push it through the hospital to collect records first thing in the morning. I would clank my way through the different departments picking up consents, lab requisitions. Sometimes they'd be unsettlingly stained; sometimes the shaky signatures would turn out to be the last thing a person ever wrote. I would hold the stacks in my arms a moment, pressing them to my chest, acknowledging that what was in those pages was privileged. That things wound up in a person's medical record that would never be shared over Christmas dinner, or in the early morning, before teeth-brushed whispers to a spouse—secrets that maybe, like mine, landed with a dull thud in the middle of a therapist's office, or between the pages of a well-hidden journal. Of course, people lie to their doctors, too, but they usually lie to themselves first.

I was making my way down one of the narrow back hallways, headed back to my office with my cart of paper secrets, when I happened by the office of one of the lab managers, a jovial older woman named Martina. We'd often chitchat as I made my rounds, and she'd often asked about what my future plans were. I was, after all, considerably younger than the other women (and it was all women) in my office. I was one of the youngest employees at the hospital, period. Naturally my presence there was a little disconcerting, but Martina took an interest in where I saw myself beyond being a literal paper pusher.

I'd mentioned a bit about my health and explained my research. I'm sure she took this as a sign that perhaps I'd go back to school, go to medical school even—and though our conversations were never long, and certainly never heavy with expectation, I did ask her if there were any opportunities that she knew of within the hospital that I wasn't yet taking full advantage of. I'd gotten certified in everything from Basic Life Support to HAZMAT ops, I sat on several committees, and I'd taken health literacy training at the Dartmouth Institute. I was generally always ready to learn something.

There was one thing I hadn't done, however, and depending on how long I kept working at the hospital, it might never come to pass that the opportunity would arise: observing an autopsy. A real cadaver—the highlight of every first-year medical student—could potentially present itself, and should it, Martina said, she'd be more than happy to put me on the pathologist's list as an observer. This announcement on her part came with the caveat that it very rarely happened that a body ended up in the morgue that needed an autopsy at our hospital. Usually they would be sent to the state crime lab.

I stood in the doorway to her office, my heart beating wildly in my ears, my leg shaking and making the cart jangle even louder, echoing down the empty, white hall.

"I didn't know we had a morgue," I said, trying not to sound too excited.

Martina gave me a knowing look. "Oh, well yeah," she said. "It's down at the end of the hall—next to the cafeteria."

I laughed, but she looked over her glasses at me. She actually wasn't kidding.

I took a short detour on the way back to my office, careening down the hall beyond the mailroom, beyond the supply closet, beyond the offshoot that opened up into the cafeteria. There, right at the end of the hallway, when I could walk no farther lest I walk straight out onto the loading dock (which I now wondered about: Had I seen them with sacks of potatoes or dead bodies?), was a practically unmarked door with a tiny sign that said "Morgue."

I tried not to get my hopes up. Martina had pointed out that it was a rather unusual thing for an autopsy to actually happen in the hospital. And besides, it wasn't something that I would have wished for—someone having to die and all. I sighed, vowing to more closely inspect the salad bar should I eat lunch at work in the coming weeks, and headed back to my office.

—⚹—

A FEW WEEKS LATER, MARTINA'S number showed up on my desk phone. When I answered, her excitement pulsed through the line before she even spoke.

"I know I said this never happens, but they're performing an autopsy this afternoon, at one o'clock. If you run up now, you'll just make it. They have to gown you up and—"

I practically shot up from my chair and looked down the row of desks to the other woman in my office who had also been on the pathologist's list.

As we jogged toward the morgue, and I realized that I didn't really know her that well. Certainly not what motivations she had for being there in that moment. What kind of conversations had she had with Martina? How long had she been waiting for this bizarre series of events to coalesce? What secrets were hidden in her medical record, between the sheets of her bed, under her skin?

The door to the morgue opened a little too easily for my sensibilities. I'd expected it to be much heavier, much more of a challenge. One minute I had been standing in the busy corridor of the hallway, among the living, and then suddenly the door closed behind me and I was in the land of the dead.

It was an extremely small space—Martina hadn't lied about that. Directly in front of where we stood were several large drawers to keep bodies chilled, but not that many. A heap of sterile blue gowns, masks, booties, and caps was just out of reach, as well as a large bin. A slender doorway led to a bathroom. Then, to the left, the door that led to the room where the autopsies took place.

An eager woman—not the pathologist, but her assistant—came out to greet us. Her cheery disposition, her pure love for her job, was a little jarring, given the otherwise still, silent air of the space. Later, I'd be grateful for her fervor. She instructed us to "suit up," showed us the bathroom, and said that we could come in "when we were ready," as the pathologist had already started the autopsy.

We hurried in, masks tightly strapped to our faces, our bodies covered from head to toe in scratchy blue, and were confronted immediately by the sights and smells that accompany these peculiar situations. Given how small the room was, although we stood with our backs pressed up against the wall (in case we fainted, so we'd slump down rather than fall face-first into an instrument tray), we were still perhaps a foot from the table on which the cadaver lay.

I have since learned who the pathologist was who conducted the autopsy, but at the time, walking into that room, I knew nothing of that person. Just one of the mysterious, masked figures who spoke little but worked quickly, arms reaching, hands tugging, heads nodding as cuts were made. The pathologist could have been anything beneath those layers of blue draper, of plastic gowns; could have been death itself for all I knew.

Much to my chagrin, no sooner had I arrived than did I realize that I had to step out to use the nook-and-cranny bathroom. I was on my period, it was heavy, and I was cramping. The words "could take five or more hours" shocked me into a certain responsibility: I'd better change my pad sooner rather than later and hope that I wouldn't pass out from blood loss later on.

I'm sure they all thought I'd left to puke rather than address my monthly exsanguination, which I was determined would not ruin the experience for me. If I bled into my pencil skirt, so be it.

When I returned, the pathologist was explaining what little they knew of the cadaver and why they were conducting an autopsy. In the event that his family ever happens across this book, I won't share any information, other than to say it was a male. This disappointed me because I desperately wanted to see a uterus in the flesh. Eventually, I'd have the opportunity to observe surgeries that would satisfy my curiosity—no dead bodies required.

I didn't have a clue what I was walking into, but I understood on some primal level that it wouldn't be anything like seeing a body at a wake or watching a *CSI* marathon. Being in the presence of death—not just death, but very fresh death—is an assault to all of your senses, even with full garb and a mask. Everything smells. The smell of blood is what you'd expect—that hot, metallic scent. The viscera itself is more earthy, almost muddy, like your backyard after a hard summer rain. Fecal matter smells the way you remember it, and of all the offensive scents, it is the least. The bile from the gallbladder, when the organ is lanced, is what made my stomach churn momentarily. Probably because bile is a fairly important component of vomit—a scent I'd become eerily familiar with thanks to my mother. If Mum had died when she half-died, when her heart gave up and greedy doctors brought her back, what would have rinsed from her digestive tract? No food, certainly. Watered-down guilt, perhaps.

There are also a lot of chemical scents, and frankly, the formaldehyde (preserving fluid) was what had me feeling light-headed. The pathologist and the technician—who mostly stayed at the foot of the table, rinsing the contents of the intestines into the sink—were so accustomed to the scents and sights and sounds that at times, both of them hummed, as if they were trimming their hedges or making a pot of tea.

Speaking of hedges: the one thing I remember the pathologist saying was in regard to the tool they used to open the ribcage. It looked like a pair of hardware store hedge clippers—and that was because *it was*.

"The single best way to remove the ribcage," the pathologist said between cracks of bone, the ribs splitting with a vulnerable crunch, "is with a set of hedge clippers from Home Depot."

The whole thing took several very long hours, but I was held in rapt attention the entire time. Suddenly those images from the textbooks that I'd been leaning over were flush and vibrant before me. I understood in a way I hadn't before that the caverns of the body are not as deep as they feel, that whatever pain I felt was closer to me than it seemed. Just beneath the surface—a little skin, a little fat, a little muscle—were these saturated, throbbing, pulsing organs that kept me alive. We hold inside of us a small ocean that gives life to the organs that give us life. Mine, like yours, sloshed about inside of me, moving and twisting with me as I'd danced and run and jumped, carrying on in their work. The patchwork of nerves and veins that had once kept this man alive, now so easily sliced with a scalpel, were such tenuous threads of life. Inside of me, a heart still beating pumped blood around my body, nerve impulses shot from my brain to my spine to the tips of my fingers twitching inside their powdered latex gloves.

The brain took the longest to be revealed—which seemed fitting to me, even then, because it is the organ that holds all the mysteries of what it means to be us.

The pathologist cut around the hairline, delicately slicing through the scalp, and folded the skin of the forehead down over the face. I almost laughed at the absurdity of it: it was like a curtain being pulled down over the final act, obscuring the star player. The man's features, the odd expression of surprise he wore, the way his sightless eyes fixated on something that fascinated him on the ceiling, were no longer relevant. I did wonder, and I still do, what that man saw last. What he thought. What he heard. What he felt.

An enormous, loudly whirring saw cut through my reverie as the pathologist worked to cut off the top of the skull. Sometimes a small hammer is used to help the lid of the skull "pop off"—it looks sort of like an ice chisel and works about the same way.

Even once the bone was removed, there were still meninges to cut through, all the while being very mindful of the delicate tissue just below. Maybe mindful, too, of the memories that haven't yet dried up.

I was somewhat surprised, after all that set-up, that the brain was simply lifted up and handed off. Turns out the brain can only be examined minimally when it's first removed; it has to soak in preservation fluid for two weeks before it will be ready to be sectioned and examined more deeply. It's because of this that autopsy reports always include, "Results pending." The brain takes the longest to examine, and many times that's where the cause of death lies. So, the other organs are returned to the body (in a bag, kind of tossed in like you'd toss a load of laundry in your hatchback on your way home from college for the weekend) before it's sewn up, so that the body is as complete as possible for burial. The brain gets sent off to the lab, taking all its mysteries with it.

That night, I couldn't sleep. Being confronted with my own mortality in such a vivid manner does that to a person, I suppose. As I lay awake, staring up at the ceiling, watching shadows dance across the room, and hoping no skeletons would run in my dreams that night, I realized I wasn't afraid of dying. What I feared was living with this kind of inescapable depth, this shaking, screaming, writhing feeling. It's that place between life and death that haunts you, as you watch someone rotting in real time, see in their eyes that last flicker of *themness*, the final mutter of life. When you watch the hull drape itself over wingback chairs and hospital beds, trying to decide whether to stay or go.

Oh, but I was teeming with life. And maybe for me, I reasoned— maybe for that man on the table who had died with his thin, bony fingers curled up as if he were making monster-hands at a little kid— living was just going to mean pain.

Still, I chewed my lip impatiently. I jiggled my foot in bed, a nervous tick. Blood whooshed in my ears. And I felt that familiar pain inside of me, on the lower right-hand side, almost comforting in its predictability, its steady presence.

What are you? I asked it, as the night enveloped me. What do you want from me?

But it was silent.

— ❦ —

WHEN I RETURNED TO DR. Wagstaff's office with my research in hand, it was a little over a year since I had seen him for the first time. He looked worried. Not because my condition had failed to improve, but because I looked like I was about to accuse him of something. I assured him that I wasn't there to question his competence—quite the opposite. I had faith that he could still help me, and now I had more information. That is, I had more clues about my case.

He waited patiently as I explained all the research I'd done regarding endometriosis—particularly, that it could be somehow related to my appendix-region pain, which had, in recent weeks, become worthy of several ER visits, including a particularly traumatic one a few weeks beforehand. That visit had been the impetus for making another appointment with Dr. Wagstaff.

The pain had been agonizing, despite the fact that Max and I had not been having sex for weeks. I couldn't even take a step without pain shooting through my abdomen as my heel touched the ground. I had gone to work in the hospital basement only to feel as though I was going to faint. My boss had sent me upstairs to the ER (extremely convenient, just an elevator ride away).

It was a small hospital, and everyone knew or at least recognized everyone else. I was also still dressed business-casual and had my badge fastened to the lapel of my blazer—a grainy photo of me with the hospital's emblem. A few nurses I knew waved as I passed through admitting, thinking I was there to collect paperwork. I practically fell onto the gurney, curling up into the fetal position, not wanting to move. I texted Max to let him know what was going on, but told him not to worry. He could come by after he got out of work if I hadn't been discharged yet.

The first nurse who came in asked me about my pain, and I must have rolled my eyes, because she looked a little bent. I explained that I'd had chronic pain for several years and my tolerance was, understandably, quite high. This pain, however, seemed louder, more exacting. I couldn't even walk without it flaring up, like a light on a dimmer switch. She said she'd come back with painkillers, but I stopped her.

"I don't want anything until I've seen the doctor," I grimaced. "I need to be able to articulate where the pain is when they ask. If you drug me up now, I won't be clear-headed enough. This isn't my first rodeo, unfortunately."

She frowned at me. "You don't want anything?"

It was my turn to frown. "Well, not until I've seen the doctor."

"It could be a while . . ."

I snorted. "No doubt. Look, I work here. I get it. I know you have to check boxes and stuff, but just say I refused. I'm not trying to be difficult, I'm just afraid that when they finally see me, if you give me all kinds of pain meds and sedatives now, I won't be able to tell them exactly where it hurts—because, see, this pain is different, and—well, I'm still trying to understand—"

"Do you want to be in pain? Do you like it?" she sneered, folding her arms.

My jaw dropped—my first thought was to tell her to go fuck herself, but I was so exhausted and nauseated that all I did was cry. She left the room without another word.

The ER doctor's note reflects my demeanor, though she didn't know exactly what had precipitated it: " . . . She is extremely frustrated and even becomes tearful."

One of the first things the doctor, a petite woman in her early thirties, did was inform me that she was going to do a vaginal exam. I must have looked grim in response, because she paused in the doorway as she headed off to ask a nurse to come assist.

"They're usually quite painful for me," I offered meekly. "Anything up there causes pain. Tampons, even. My boyfriend and I don't have sex anymore . . ."

She nodded and went to fetch the nurse—the same one from before. They put my legs up in stirrups without looking at me. I took a

deep breath and tried to relax, having become quite skilled at meta-
physically leaving my body to avoid the pain. The doctor went to
insert the speculum and I cried out, my body contorting involuntarily
up from the table. The nurse gasped, her mouth now open enough to
eat her words from earlier.

"I'm okay, I'm okay," I said, my breath unsteady. "Just get it over
with."

The doctor looked at me a moment, then tried again—I screamed,
tears streaming down my face, and felt a warm hand take mine. When
I opened my eyes, I saw the nurse looking down at me apologetically.

Of course they'd found nothing and sent me home, but when I
noticed my own ER document in a stack of paperwork in medical
records when I went back to work the following week, what jumped
out at me from the page was that the emergency room physician had
noted me as being anxious to the point of tears.

Yeah, no shit, I thought as I ripped staples out of charts with a
little more effort than was strictly necessary. *I can't eat, sleep, dance,
walk, or fuck. Wouldn't you cry, too, if it happened to you?*

When I presented my findings to Dr. Wagstaff, he didn't know
quite what to make of it—or of me.

"You're either brilliant or the most well-educated hypochondriac
I've ever met," he said, shaking his head lightly. He agreed to do another laparoscopy; at the very least he could remove my appendix so
that I wouldn't have to worry about it. Aside from that, he warned
me that if the procedure turned up nothing he'd have to discharge me
from his practice. There just wasn't anything else he could do.

AT THE BEGINNING, MAX TRIED to bolster my spirits during my
many days and nights of pain and the endless string of doctor's visits.
I remember him sitting next to me as I sipped on pink contrast dye before a CT scan, saying, "StrawBarium Pink Drink is what they should
call it"—and I had genuinely laughed at that. But after several rounds
of this with no signs of improvement, he had grown frustrated. He
was twenty-something years old; he wanted to have a normal life,
party with his friends, and have a cute girlfriend he could show off.
I think he was at first disappointed that I never felt well enough to

join him. Then, he began to resent me for it. He began to feel that his needs weren't being met sexually, and he was absolutely right—they were not. I was not a good partner. I couldn't possibly be one in the state I was in. Of course, my sexual needs weren't being met either, but no one really asked me if I was sexually frustrated. The prevailing theory seemed to be that I had so much pain with sex because I didn't like it.

I offered to stay at his parents' house to recover, which would essentially get him off the hook. He wouldn't be stuck having to help me get up to go to the bathroom, or bring me tea, or accidentally knee me in my tender stomach in the night. His parents had a guest bedroom that was a very short limping distance to the upstairs bathroom. I could stay there relatively unobtrusively until I was well enough to go home and look after myself.

The night before my second surgery, I washed my skin with the antiseptic soap the hospital had given me, staying in the shower at his parents' house a lot longer than I needed to in order to get clean. I was trying to cleanse myself of something else: the pervasive thoughts that maybe I was just making this all up. Maybe all of this was in my head.

Max, and his parents, knew so much about my childhood. They knew how hard it had been, and I know they felt for me, wished that it could have been different. Still, they marveled at what I had achieved. Financial independence, for one. I owned a car, though it was a beater, and made sure all our bills were paid on time. More importantly, that *my* bills were paid. I had close to $10,000 in medical debt racked up by then, not to mention student loans that were coming out of deferment. I'd hoped to invest what little I could save so that I could begin to put away money for my brother, as I was to assume legal guardianship of him when I turned thirty (the magic age at which I, my parents, and the legal system had assumed I'd have my shit together enough to do so).

Although I hadn't been able to go back to school, which was what I really wanted to do, I'd gotten a perfectly respectable job with benefits, sick days, and paid vacation. I had friends with college degrees who had been unable to wrangle that in the economy they'd graduated into. I think Max's parents had started to expect that Max and I would get married, and if it hadn't been for my waning health, and the stress it had put on our relationship, that may have happened. As Jane had predicted years before, I'd learned a great deal about myself through my relationship with Max. I'd matured emotionally in ways that allowed me to trust, and to become comfortable with being vulnerable once in a while, and I had certainly acquired a little more self-esteem. I still became considerably agitated about people throwing up, though, and I still hadn't managed to tame my zeal about whatever weird new thing I'd learned about in a given week. I wouldn't even dare hazard a guess as to how many hours of TED-style presentations Max sat through after I learned about the "random article" button on Wikipedia.

My head was already full of so much, I thought as I stepped out of the shower, sinking down to sit on the edge of the tub. I couldn't imagine that my brain had the bandwidth necessary to construct some kind of elaborate medical crisis. Maybe if it had only lasted a few weeks, I could have accepted it as some kind of glitch in the matrix, but it had been going on for years now. I sat there dripping, growing cold as the fog dissipated from the room, and I was paralyzed with fear: What if I was lying, to everyone—even myself? What if the pain wasn't real at all, what if it never had been? Had Dr. Wagstaff been right all along? Had the trauma from my childhood, which I had diligently worked to resolve, which I had taken copious antidepressants to dull the ache of, somehow escaped my brain and taken up residence in my bones? Could anguish live, truly, in your actual heart, and not just your metaphysical heart? Was my body shutting down in response to years of being unwanted and unloved, of being alone and unaccounted for? Had my brain succeeded in convincing my body that it had no right to live? Could emotional pain actually cause your physical body to slowly rot away, like some sort of dramatic, psychological consumption? Was I really losing my mind rather than my body? Was I a Freudian hysteric with an iPhone?

All night I tossed and turned in bed, the heaviness of my body's ache feeling as though it would send me down, down, down through the mattress and the bed frame, and the floorboards, through the cellar and into the ground, until I settled six feet below.

Max and his mother took me to the hospital early the next morning. Only one of them could come into pre-op with me, and although

I reached for Max, there was a part of me that would have preferred his mom. Less specifically, a mom. I was scared shitless, once again, and Max had grown distant.

Earlier in the week, he'd told me that he thought it was only fair that he got to sleep with other girls while I recovered. I was aghast and asked him if he no longer intended to be monogamous. He immediately scoffed, saying that monogamy wasn't a fair expectation given the circumstances. I tried to see his point. I felt ashamed enough that I had failed to be a giving partner, and part of me was just so exhausted by living that the thought of him getting his needs met elsewhere was almost a weight lifted from my shoulders. Except that I have always been a girl of principles. Even as a little girl, I'd had a stringent sense of right and wrong. If we had agreed to be monogamous, then we should be monogamous. If he no longer wanted that . . . well, maybe we should break up. Neither of us really wanted that, but we were beginning to feel the necessity for change. We couldn't go on as we had been. Or at least he couldn't.

Then again, he wasn't tucked into a hospital bed, attached to an IV pole, putting his fate into the hands of an anesthesiologist who made awkward, off-color dad-jokes. Unlike the first surgery I'd had years before, I wasn't awake when they took me into the OR. The sedative knocked me out midsentence while we were all still in pre-op.

When I came to in recovery several hours later, I felt different before I even opened my eyes. There was definitely an absent feeling in my abdomen—a sensation I had come to understand intellectually the previous year, when my best friend Hillary had given birth to her son, one social event at which I had been present.

She'd had an emergency C-section at the last minute, but certainly she, too, had experienced a distinct feeling of, "Wow, there's not a baby inside me anymore." Having never been pregnant myself, I guess I can't claim it's at all the same thing, but I was startled to wake up and have something that I had become so accustomed to, a familiar feeling inside my body—even when it was, at times, a real fucker—having completely vanished.

The nurse noticed I was coming around and started feeding me ice chips. My eyes struggled to focus on his face, but when I'd centered myself, I had only one question.

"What was it?"

He and the other recovery nurses exchanged a look between them, and he kind of shook his head in disbelief.

"You were right. It was your appendix."

It wasn't just that it was my appendix, though. It would need to be confirmed with pathology (which it was), but it appeared that the infection had been subacute and chronic, meaning that, as I'd hypothesized, it had been going on for quite some time. The appendix was extremely long and densely adherent. Adhesions, in and of themselves—particularly in the bowel—can certainly cause a person pain and suffering. On top of that, the portion of my intestine from whence the appendix emerges, the cecum, was "floppy," and not attached to my abdominal wall as it should have been. This abnormality, sometimes called "mobile cecum," probably occurs during fetal development. But, because the cecum can move, that means that, so long as there's an appendix at the end of it, that can move too. When Dr. Wagstaff found it, it was retrocecal—behind the cecum. That positioning had probably been part of the reason why the whole mess hadn't shown up on any scan.

I stared at the hot, white ceiling, not yet able to move or really say anything else. I had never wanted to be right, only to be well. Dr. Wagstaff, admittedly, didn't know what would happen next. Maybe I'd have lingering problems, or maybe I'd feel better. There wasn't a lot of research on it, and the majority of doctors didn't believe it was even possible. Even among those who regarded it as a possibility, the infrequency of the condition in medical literature implied that few doctors would see it in their careers. Dr. Wagstaff half-joked that he should write a paper. After he left, I turned to Max and said, "If he does, I think I should at least get to coauthor it. I did all the research." I'd never defended a thesis or even gained enough credits for a degree, but I'd completed enough research to save my own life, which had to count for something.

In any case, I would have a story to tell myself about resilience and determination, about advocating for my inner, visceral truth. Maybe it wasn't bound in leather and sitting in a university library or hanging framed in a corner office, but the scars on my abdomen would do.

I had managed to vanquish one pain from my body, cast it out like a pacing spirit, but I mistook that minor exorcism for salvation.

Pain was not done with me, and though I felt prepared to stare it down, it would find ways to lurk in the shadows, unnoticed, until it decided to angrily beat its wings again.

IN THE END, IT REALLY didn't matter how much I loved Max, just the same as it had never mattered how much I wanted not to be sick. When we finally went our separate ways, I felt responsible. The continued intimation, on the part of doctors and society, that my inability to engage in sexual intercourse was somehow by my choosing, that it was something deeper than parts that didn't work in accordance with my desires, only made me question myself and my role in the relationship.

If I was truly in love with him and attracted to him, wouldn't I put up with whatever pain our intimacy caused? Indeed, I had, for quite some time by this point. I had buried my face in a pillow feigning pleasure when I was crying from pain. When I finally reached the point where I couldn't lie about it anymore, my truth became a broken record that sounded like an excuse. It must have sounded like I wasn't attracted to him anymore, and that I didn't love him. But relationships are complex because humans are complex. He moved away to battle his own demons. I have since realized that's the only way it could have been—because I was one of them.

I stayed in the apartment we'd shared together because I wasn't ready to leave. I had never stayed in one place for so long, and even though memories hovered thick in the air, after some time had passed, they cleared like a fog. The ones that lingered I could gently coax down with a broom or some incense.

I stayed in touch with his parents, since we still orbited one another in the same community. I found that I missed them in ways I could not miss Max, and that there were times when their loss was heavier than his.

Several years later, Max came to visit, and we met for coffee at the same café where we'd met half a decade earlier. He looked almost exactly the same—his hair a little shorter, maybe, his voice a little tentative, unsure. But he was more centered. On an even keel, he would have said, being the sailor. As we talked, the sky unleashed a downpour.

We had become, as time allows, very different people. But we found relief, and a little delight, in those split seconds when our eyes lit up at the same joke, or we recalled some shared memory. He was getting ready for a late summer trek into the wilderness with his parents, escaping from his new city life for a week. I accompanied him to a sporting goods store in town so he could get a rain slicker. We sat down in some very small folding chairs, next to where the pop tents were displayed in the carpeted, interior woods. It was a strange place to spill our guilt to one another, but it was also kind of the perfect place.

We each carried guilt regarding the other, but we managed to begin the process of absolving it—right there next to those Coleman tents. When we stepped outside, he with a brand new jacket, it had stopped raining. It was inexplicably sunny and beautiful as we went our separate ways.

I went back to my apartment alone. There had always been bits of him around, dust of his in the air. I slowly reclaimed the space, made the mess my own. I let the good memories float unbound around me. Every experience that reaffirmed I had known happiness, and had been capable of love, was worth grasping for.

CHAPTER 7

I began to have a smaller regard for the ability of doctors
than I ever had before, and a greater one for myself.

—Nellie Bly, *Ten Days in the Madhouse*

IN HER MEMOIR *GIVING UP THE GHOST*, Hilary Mantel recounts her experience of being diagnosed with endometriosis in the late 1970s. Her journey, like mine, began when she was nineteen, and she had a hysterectomy when she was twenty-seven. The stories of so many women I've talked to echo hers. You'd think that in the forty-some years that have elapsed, something would have changed, and a woman my age wouldn't be having the same experience that Mantel, now in her sixties, had decades ago. I cringed reading passages from her memoir because the feeling of recognition angered me. I was angry for her, that she'd suffered, but also angry that not much seems to have changed.

"He calls me Little Miss Neverwell," she wrote of one of her doctors. "I am angry. I don't like being given a name. It's too much like power over me."

Mantel, like many other patients still today, took the diagnosis of endometriosis to her physician (okay, several of them) after reading about it in a medical textbook. But this only came after years of being misdiagnosed with what she recalls as "stress, caused by over-ambition," for which she was overmedicated with tranquilizers.

She mentions frequently that she probably would have been better off saying nothing at all of her physical symptoms—which were always seen as psychosomatic complaints. "The more I said that I had a physical illness, the more they said I had a mental illness," she wrote. "The more I questioned the nature, the reality of the mental illness, the more I was found to be in denial, deluded."

An accomplished novelist, Mantel was once told by a psychiatrist to stop writing. I, for one, am glad that she didn't, if only because she did write that memoir (a bit reluctantly, it seems, if you take in her self-deprecation throughout). Endometriosis, she noted, had a reputation for plaguing high-achieving women, addressing the phenomenon with a single, biting sentence: "It used to be fashionable to call endometriosis the 'career woman's disease': the implication being, there now, you callous bitch, see what you get if you put off breeding and put your own ambitions first?"

As a woman with endo still seeking information and treatment in the early 1980s, Mantel endured the height of this particular perception of endometriosis. But such descriptions seemed to have a somewhat similar bent as early as the 1930s: American physician Joe Vincent Meigs, for example, found endometriosis to be the result of women delaying childbearing too long. Those who went against nature became the victims of nature's wiles.

Comparing women to apes seemed perfectly reasonable to Meigs, who wagered that female apes probably didn't menstruate much at all, because they began having babies as soon as they were able and didn't stop "until [they were] dead." He added: "As women have the same physiology [as apes] it must be wrong to put off childbearing until 14 to 20 years of menstrual life have passed." One wonders if Meigs actually knew any women.

Meigs also suggested that endometriosis was primarily limited to the upper echelons of society—as these women seemed to have "a difference in attitude toward childbearing"—and basically, that they should just stop whining and have babies if they wanted to be cured. He was also eager to remind his colleagues to only encourage reproduction among their higher-class patients, however—and never those in the lower classes. The eugenics vibe is real here, and it was Meigs's accounts that laid the foundation for decades of research that focused on endometriosis as a disease of well-educated white women. Specifically, a disease of fertility, above all else.

A January 2017 study reported that one in ten British women experienced painful sex—and the majority of the women experiencing it were in middle age (the second-largest group was younger, ages sixteen to twenty-four). The data was gathered over a period of two years from nearly 7,000 women in the United Kingdom. Not surprisingly, the findings indicated that there are myriad reasons why a woman may experience painful sex. The main limitation of the study—as is true of most existing surveys that attempt to capture data about pain—was the inability to firmly denote causality. It seems likely that much of what women self-reported was interdependent: that is, each individual's experience with painful sex is ultimately determined by many variables, a few of which they have little to no control over (their partner, a physician, etc.). About 2 percent of the women in the study reported painful sex that occurred frequently and that had been plaguing them for longer than six months, causing them a great deal of distress. Researchers referred to this category as "morbid painful sex."

The study had primarily surveyed sexually active women who were part of a much larger cohort—but there were some women who said they were no longer sexually active *because of* the pain during sex. They reported avoidance, fear of pain, and lack of interest as the reasons why they were no longer sexually active. Fully 62 percent of women who reported experiencing painful sex said they were no longer interested in having it, compared to 31 percent of women who did not report painful sex. Although these women did self-report their experience for the survey, whether they had been able to report their pain to others with any degree of success (partners, physicians) is less clear. The researchers pointed to other studies in their conclusion, so as not to let this point be lost: "Only a fraction of women affected by genital pain disorders ever receive an official diagnosis: 1.4% in a study of women meeting criteria for vulvodynia [vulvar pain]. In a previous paper . . . we reported that less than half of women with morbid symptoms of sexual pain had sought professional help in the last year. Among those who do seek treatment, negative experiences are common, including invalidated concerns,

not receiving a formal diagnosis, and being given treatment perceived as ineffective."

⁓🎗⊕

IN THE MONTHS AFTER MAX and I broke up, an isolated sexual experience proved to me that it was never that I had fallen out of love
with him. Nor had I ever stopped being attracted to him—something
was *very* wrong inside my body.

Not that I planned it, but when the opportunity presented itself
to have sex with a man who was in every conceivable way Max's
opposite, I recognized that it would provide me with invaluable information. In the moment, admittedly, I was not quite that clinical
about it: I just liked the guy a lot. His name was William, and unlike
a lot of people named William, he didn't go by a nickname. It wasn't
pretentious at all—he was the least pretentious, most easygoing person you'd ever chance to meet. For whatever reason, he was William
in toto. Had things gone differently that night, I would have no doubt
seriously dated him, and who knows where it might have gone?

William happened to be in town one weekend a couple of months
after Max and I broke up. He knew both of us pretty well, and I think
that, like many people in our lives at that time, he thought Max and
I would be together for the long haul. Knowing about the split, he
dropped by to say hello and see how things were going. We chatted,
and although I can't exactly tell you how we got there, he turned to
me with a rather sweet apprehensiveness. He had apparently harbored
feelings for me for quite some time. Not that he intended to capitalize
on the recent breakup just then, but should I ever be interested . . .

"We could have sex now," I shrugged. He didn't say anything at
first, and I thought maybe my forwardness had been a little much.
I have never been what you might call subtle. When I looked up to
where he was standing in the doorway, he was beaming at me.

"I've, uh . . . it's just . . ." he squeaked. "I've fantasized about this
for a long time."

"Oh," I said softly, flattered and vaguely terrified by the revelation. "So, um. Do you have a condom?" I don't generally make it
a practice of crushing men's dreams, but as sheer panic crossed his
face, my heart sank.

"Hold on," he said, fumbling for his keys. "I'll just—I'll run to the store just, uh. Just wait here and I'll—"

He disappeared out into the hallway, and a few minutes later, I heard his engine rev. I recognized that, if I should want to change my mind, I now had the opportunity to do so. But I didn't. For the next ten minutes or so I sat calmly on the bed. His condom run completed in record time, I heard him powering up the stairs—ripping into the box as he did—and I found myself unexpectedly charmed.

The experience of being intimate with him bore no resemblance to anything I'd become familiar with, but that hardly meant it was bad. If anything, as he gently reveled in his fantasy of me come to life, I found myself earnestly hoping that it would be different in the most profound of ways: that it wouldn't hurt.

I intuited from his attentiveness, his thoughtfulness, the sort of gentle reverence he had for the moment and for me, that he was a good lover. I was somewhat startled to realize that an hour had gone by and he was in no hurry—just pleasantly sedate, with a bit of a doofy, disbelieving grin. By the time he actually penetrated me, I'd been enjoying his joy and my own sort of pleasant surprise that I'd all but forgotten I had been worried about the pain I'd come to expect.

I thought for a brief moment before we began having intercourse that maybe, just maybe, it wasn't going to hurt. So when that same familiar pain arose and displaced my pleasure, stole it from me, I was stricken. Whereas before I had been disappointed, embarrassed, guilt-ridden, and sexually frustrated, this time what filled me was exhaustive rage. Then, a sickening fear.

Afterward, I did not want William to stay, but not because of anything he'd done or not done. I just didn't want him to hear me crying in the shower. I didn't want him to feel the sticky warmth of blood on the sheets in the night. I didn't want to wake to see him the next morning, knowing there was no way to explain that he'd hurt me, but the fault was mine.

As the months turned to years, I continued to be confused by the fact that although I was capable of sexual arousal, and, theoretically, enjoyed a lot of what sex had to offer, it always came to a sudden, wounding halt once any kind of significant penetration occurred. I was also well aware that orgasms—which cause mild uterine contractions—left me with a heavy, nauseating ache for at least a day. Even orgasms that resulted from clitoral stimulation alone would cause that post-heat ache. Sometimes it was actually worse, and lasted longer—I assume because the orgasms were better.

As I attempted to construct some kind of meaningful discourse about this experience, I began to consider how my analysis of my pain—however thorough—had always been criticized by others for one glaring flaw: a small sample size. It was bad enough that my sex life had become all but reduced to a clinical trial, but the constant rhetoric of "you just haven't had enough sex with enough people" from a few female friends confounded me. And it was bad enough when male doctors disregarded my pain, but when women did—especially women I considered friends or mentors—I almost felt betrayed. What if I didn't want to gather men like specimens? Wasn't it enough that I had been engaged in a consensual sexual relationship with two men, both of whom I cared about deeply, men whose company I enjoyed? Wasn't it enough that I had wanted to be able to have sex with them without the need for an official investigation or some kind of epidemiological survey? What difference did it make whether it hurt to have sex with ten men I didn't care about or one man that I did?

I'm sure it was an attempt to be helpful, and it wasn't as though this was something that had been repeated to me by every person I encountered. It didn't have to be—once it got into my head, I had to chew it over. Eventually, though, I abandoned my computations in favor of my feelings—not particularly scientific, but not something I could altogether discount. The implication seemed to be that I was in pain because I was sexually inexperienced, which kind of missed the point as far as I was concerned: it wasn't the sex I found confusing, it was the pain that resulted from engaging in it. The fine details might change, but the mechanics of heterosexual intercourse would be the same. Therefore the number of sexual partners should not matter.

What if a more Freudian interpretation was necessary, then? Could it be that, beneath the implication that I just didn't "get" sex yet, there was this undercurrent of doubt, on the part of doctors and friends, in my ability to interpret pain? And perhaps the doubters were correct: I was misinterpreting pleasure as something unpleasant, perhaps even subconsciously? Or consciously attempting to evade the physical aspects of my sexuality? Could I be using my pain for some other as-yet-to-be-determined reason, perhaps as a tool of manipulation? These theories seemed a lot more complex and nuanced than my problem when it came to sex: it hurt.

Despite my efforts to argue the contrary, I never seemed to be able to articulate properly that the pain was irrespective of my state of arousal, my interest, or my skill. It existed even in the absence of a partner—a fact I was rarely able to bring up, as I found people were perfectly happy to gossip about sex so long as we didn't traipse into the wanton world of masturbation. Even doctors wouldn't ask; I always offered the information because I found it startling and distressing and figured it was therefore relevant. I was the primary source of data for the investigation into my condition, and yet it often felt like the data I presented was questioned by others as unreliable. Thus, I questioned myself.

Eventually, I could no longer put energy into the inquisition; nor did I have the wherewithal to grieve its loss. Of all the demands of humanity that I was struggling with, there were things of greater importance on the hierarchy of needs than sex that I had to deal with. I never made a decision to be celibate. I am still rendered weak-kneed by attractive men I encounter in my travels. I am not, nor have I ever been, "frigid" or "prudish." I am, however, resigned: a woman's sexual pleasure is rarely anyone's priority, not even her own.

IN HER REVIEW OF LITERATURE on endometriosis back in 2003, Carolyn Carpan explored how the media—women's magazines, national news outlets, and so on—had presented endometriosis to the general public. In recent years, as several high-profile celebrities have come out as having endometriosis, the word has occasionally popped up more. A simple Google Trends search from 2004 to the present shows a fairly steady interest, but the spikes can be correlated to those announcements. The word inexplicably reached peak popularity in September 2004—the only article I could find published that month was from the BBC, which mentioned endo but was actually about a cannabis-like chemical that US researchers believed could be important to a normal pregnancy. In other months of 2004, the BBC also had several other articles about endometriosis, but overall, the archive search of news turned up just three pages of results.

Using Google's Ngram Viewer, however, we can look at the presence of the word "endometriosis" in English-language texts over a much longer period of time—several centuries, in fact. If we set our parameters to begin in the 1800s and end with the present day, the upward trend is obvious. Meigs's work in the 1930s seems to have started a slight upward trend over the next decade, which leveled off for awhile in the 1950s—which is not surprising, considering that women in that decade were somewhat notoriously subdued by a mix of "uppers" and "downers," and their gynecological experiences, such as childbearing, often occurred behind a veil of "twilight sleep." After World War II, "pep pills"—amphetamines that had commonly been handed out to soldiers—made their way back to the home front. They were marketed to America's housewives as a cure for depression, with the added benefit of weight loss. But the amphetamines would keep them awake at night, especially at higher doses. Furthermore, once a woman began to develop a tolerance, she'd need something to help her sleep. That's where barbiturate sedatives came in. At one point, there was so much pharmaceutical competition that one company actually developed a drug that mixed a barbiturate (amobarbital) with an amphetamine (dextroamphetamine). It was called Dexamyl, and it was sold as a diet drug, an antianxiety drug, and an antidepressant. Other, similar drugs followed, such as a mix of amphetamines and phenobarbital.

The use of these drugs reached epidemic proportions throughout the 1950s and 1960s, but it wasn't particularly illicit. Women experienced a pharmaceutical whirlwind when they went into the hospital to have a baby, for example. Many women alive today, our mothers and grandmothers, probably gave birth under the influence of a cocktail of drugs, such as morphine and scopolamine. A woman would be given an injection even before she was in full-on labor; it was designed to keep her aware enough to take commands from the doctor when she needed to deliver, but also gave her total amnesia about the experience. Which, not infrequently, involved her being tied down to the bed. Many women from that era can remember going into the hospital, getting a shot, and waking up with a clean, pink, sleeping baby being placed into their arms. But there were also plenty of women who woke up to discover they'd had a C-section, or some other intervention to which they had not strictly consented, because they'd been unable to deliver naturally—and it may have been that the drugs compromised their ability to push effectively. Make no mistake: the twilight sleep protocols weren't about making childbirth easier for women—it was about making it easier for doctors.

I'm certain that women were suffering from endometriosis in the 1950s and 1960s—but I suspect that many of them were self-medicating, and "grinning and bearing it" when they weren't, as was the expectation of their husbands, families, and doctors.

From the 1960s to the mid-1970s, there was a pretty steep decline in references to endometriosis—which seems peculiar to me, because it was the height of the feminist movement. From the 1980s to the present day, however, there has been a marked and steady upward trend, probably aided in part by the ubiquity of the Internet.

As Carpan pointed out in her review, though, just seeing the word more doesn't necessarily correlate to a greater understanding of the disease. If anything, the way endometriosis has largely been depicted by the media has lent itself to the stereotype presented to Mantel, that endometriosis is "a career woman's disease." It's not fair to blame the press entirely for this characterization—after all, reporters are only citing research. For their quotations, they're looking to doctors, a disproportionate number of whom are middle-aged white men who are somehow experts on a disease they will never have.

The position of these articles, even if they are admirably researched, is very much in the service of the intended audience. What seems to be consistent across the various genres of media, however, is the focus on endometriosis as primarily a disease of fertility. The women interviewed are always devastated that they have become, or may yet become, infertile. The doctors encourage young women with endometriosis to get pregnant as soon as possible—even claiming that it may "cure" their disease. Catherine Kohler Riessman, a research professor in the Department of Sociology at Boston College and an emerita professor at Boston University, has written extensively on the medicalization of women's health. She suggests that this particular framing of endometriosis comes from physicians' re-inforcement of gendered, social norms through the pathologizing of something deemed abnormal—such as a childless woman.

I have often felt that my explicit intention to be childless had a direct and exceedingly negative impact on my diagnosis and treat-ment, especially because it preceded any problems I had with my reproductive system. My family often recalled how, when my brother was still a baby—so I couldn't have been more than four years old—I announced one day that I didn't want to go to heaven because "the baby Jesus probably cries all the time."

Prior to the first surgery with Dr. Paulson, she'd made a point to impress an awareness upon me that any procedure involving my reproductive organs could conceivably pose a threat to my fertility. I could not sincerely behave as though the loss of my fertility was my biggest concern in that moment; nor could I do so after I found out she hadn't removed the cyst, because the surgery could have been injurious to the fallopian tube to which it was attached. Before that surgery—and any surgery I'd ever have—I made it quite clear that even if it meant I'd lose an ovary, I expected whatever needed to be dealt with to be dealt with. Because even if I had wanted children, I certainly didn't want them at nineteen, or even at twenty-three. Even my mild attempts to entertain the idea of childbearing were never something I could envision happening before my mid-thirties, and that was a solid decade away. I tried to explain this to Dr. Paulson, to Dr. Wagstaff, to Jane—to anyone who would have listened, really. And inevitably, I would wince with a little half-smile and offer a half-hearted, "Maybe I'd like to have a baby when I'm older . . ." in order to placate them, because expressing a preference toward childlessness is apparently quite the faux pas.

The things that actually did concern me—the pain, the nausea, the complete loss of everything that I loved and that made me happy (food, dance, sex)—didn't seem to carry the kind of weight that con-cerns about my fertility did. How, I wonder, did the doctors expect me to get pregnant if I couldn't have sex? What if I had said, "Okay, fine, I'll have a baby—but how, pray tell, shall I go about it when sex is excruciatingly painful and I can't tolerate penetration long enough to be fertilized?"

Why wasn't it enough that I was a young woman who wanted to be sexually active, but couldn't be? Did the fact that I wanted sexual pleasure, intimacy with a partner—dare I say, fun?—without the responsibility of procreating make me somehow less than the women who did? Did people, medical professionals and others, really think that I'd asked for it, somehow? That endometriosis was my punishment for wanting a career? For wanting sex and pleasure? For rejecting the biological imperative to procreate? Maybe it wasn't quite so overt, but, as Carpan discovered through her review of the literature, maybe it doesn't even have to be. These beliefs are pervasive, but in the same quiet, pernicious way that endometriosis is. The way ovarian cancers are. Even the diseases that befall women are silent, controlled, unseen.

At least that's how they're characterized in medical textbooks, largely because those who have historically done the characterizing are men. If women had been their equals in the fields of science and medicine, if they could have contributed clinically and academically during the formative years of those disciplines, I suspect the characterizations would have been quite different. Although a male physician could quite easily, and convincingly, assert that ovarian cancer was "silent," if you were to really listen to women who have had ovarian cancer speak, you'd find that it wasn't so much that the disease process was silent—but that they were. Conditions that seem to lurk unnoticed in a woman's body go unnoticed by others because, for one thing, they are an assumed part of womanhood, and, for another, women are taught to keep those pains private. I've often found it curious that when a woman is suffering, her competence is questioned, but when a man is suffering, he's humanized. It's a gender stereotype that hurts both men and women, though it lends itself to the question of why there is a proclivity in health care, and in society, to deny female pain.

The most oft-cited study directly addressing this issue, "The Girl Who Cried Pain," was published in 2001. Authors Diane E. Hoffmann and Anita J. Tarzian open with the passage from the Bible where God says women will bear children and it will hurt A LOT. I knew the quote, but I had never really considered the next phrase, which is, " . . . yet your desire will be for your husband, and he shall rule over you." Which kind of makes it sound like a damned if you do, damned if you don't situation. Was the intent all along for sex to hurt for women, even if they were having the kind of sex that the Bible says God is okay with?

After the introduction, Hoffmann and Tarzian drop a real whopper of a statement: postoperation, women are more likely to be given sedatives for pain, whereas men are more likely to be given pain medication. There are several logical explanations for this, my favorite of which is the idea that men are naturally so stoic that if they say they aren't in pain, they must be in pain. Women, meanwhile, just complain a lot. Men were more likely to receive pain medication postoperatively than women following heart bypass surgery, for example. Women were more likely to receive sedatives; but even when women did receive pain medication, they got considerably less of it than the men (even after accounting for differences in weight, which affects dosing). If you extrapolate a little, it's pretty easy to see that women were given sedatives because they were perceived to be anxious more than they were perceived to be in pain. Such findings apply even in children. One study showed that boys were more likely to be given codeine postoperatively than girls; the girls, meanwhile, were given acetaminophen—that is, Tylenol.

Men are expected to be stoic in the face of pain, which is bad enough for them—but their dedication to that stoicism only makes it harder for women to have their pain taken seriously. Women, it seems, have to prove that they are as sick as men before they will be given the same level of care. The harder a man pushes himself to deny his own pain, the harder a woman will have to fight to have her pain acknowledged.

Although it's true that men may be pressured into stoicism socially, when I think of stoicism in the face of pain, I think of women. Admittedly, this is anecdotal evidence, but from talking to my women friends, I've observed that whenever a guy gets a cold, he becomes a weeny, staying in bed for three days with a runny nose. The women, meanwhile, get up and go to work with fevers of 102. It's not always the case, of course: my father practically never missed a day of work in his entire life, save for the half-day off he took when he had some teeth pulled and couldn't drive, while my mother was so ill that she never worked.

Most of the women I know, especially those who have children, couldn't be stopped from taking on their daily schedules by anything less than a complete limb amputation. Even then, I'm sure they'd just stuff it into a diaper bag and carry on. I wish I could say I was being entirely facetious here, but I'm not, and history has my back on this. Women have been laboring through their labor for centuries—only pausing momentarily during the bountiful harvest to push out a baby, popping its squalling mouth onto their ample bosom and continuing to shuck corn. No one else in the field probably even batted an eye, further reinforcing the idea that female pain is an evolutionary constant.

All of this relates to that old mandate in 1993 when researchers figured out that men and women had different drug responses. The one that said: actually, you have to include women in your clinical research—*sorry*. Things began to change with the NIH Revitalization Act passed that year. And yet, since women were excluded from clinical research for such a long time, it only makes sense that we would still have more data on men. More data on men that is largely still being analyzed in medical journals by men, and then being read by men. Because, you know, despite passage of the NIH act, we're not quite at the point where women are dominating clinical research or medicine.

Two terms that are necessary to understand when talking about pain, and that Hoffmann and Tarzian differentiated beautifully in their paper, are "threshold" and "tolerance." Pain tolerance is talked about frequently, especially in the context of sex differences. Tolerance refers to the point at which a person in pain can no longer tolerate it. Their pain threshold refers to the level at which they first begin to consciously experience pain. We talk a lot about a person's pain tolerance but far less frequently about their pain threshold. One might assume that if a person has a very high pain threshold—that is, they don't begin to feel pain for a long time compared to others in the same situation—they may also, then, have a very high pain tolerance. Or the inverse: that someone who has a low pain threshold has, too, a very low tolerance for pain.

I'd say that's probably an easy conclusion to reach, but one that lacks the nuances of how human beings actually work. How they adapt to the situation when pain becomes present, and then when it becomes constant. I'm sure we all know a story of a woman, a friend or coworker, or our own mothers, who went into labor only to continue on about their day. They cleaned the house or ran an errand, pausing occasionally as a contraction momentarily swelled. Other women may not begin to feel the punch of labor until it has progressed much more, at which time they clamor for an epidural. I've known women in both camps.

When I first got sick, I had been dancing on a full-time schedule for at least a year, and while I would admit to a low pain threshold, my tolerance, once I was in pain, was relatively high. I could perceive pain astutely, perhaps because dancers come to understand parts of their bodies with a kind of intimacy most people go a lifetime without knowing. I could feel the moment before pain started in some muscles in my legs.

I anticipated it, braced for it even, whenever my bad ankle was required to carry its weight. I wouldn't be surprised to hear that many dancers, athletes, movers in other methods, have this sort of sixth sense for pain. The pain I experienced when I fell ill, however, was so abrupt that I received no such premonition. There was no warning. And what went unappreciated, I think, was that I actually had quite a high degree of tolerance for the pain I was in. I couldn't seem to explain to anyone that I actually wasn't terribly distressed about being in pain—pain became kind of a normal part of my life. Rather, I was frightened because it was a new pain, one I had never felt before, and the symptoms associated with it made the whole experience something I couldn't make sense of. I wasn't afraid of the pain, necessarily—I was afraid of what was causing it.

There were certain pains that I could dance through. Certain pains I'd learned to live through, and with, that I came to know in early childhood. Hunger, for one, was a pain that I knew well, until I became numb to it. I understood that pain was a language of the body, but that my body wasn't always trying to communicate an emergency.

Sometimes it was just saying, I'm stretching, I'm growing, I'm alive. If it was crying out, a shrill "enough! enough!," I'd usually ask it to press on a little more. Sometimes it would sigh, submitting to the movement, and sometimes it would resist: "No, I really mean it!"

And I would become bitterly subservient to its need for rest. The pain I had come to live with did not allow me to ask it anything.

But I am not the first woman—nor, sadly, am I bound to be the last—who has made a life as the mistress of pain. I've spent many a late night wide awake in bed wondering how far back it goes, this legacy. Did our Neanderthal ancestors have a way to communicate "No, it's fine—I'm fine—really!" Are these behavioral mechanisms of avoidance and denial intrinsically female? Some research has implied that yes, women are more likely to cope through emotionally focused strategies, whereas men take a more direct, problem-solving kind of approach. Though I would question whether it's really intrinsic or if it's just that men haven't had to devise the kind of coping mechanisms that women have, because their pain is taken seriously and remedied as soon as it becomes apparent.

In reviewing the work in "The Girl Who Cried Pain" for the first time, years ago in the hospital library, I wondered if maybe I'd been talking about my pain in such a way that it invalidated me. Women tend to contextualize their pain when describing it, whether to a medical professional or a friend: they discuss how it has impacted their ability to work, their day-to-day lives, their relationships. Men typically do not provide this context, instead just stating the facts.

The next time I saw a doctor, I attempted to do it the manly way, and state my symptoms without providing any emotional context. What was interesting was that the doctor asked for it: Was the pain bad enough to negatively impact my ability to work? I caved and reverted back to "emotional context," but I wondered: Why did it matter? If I had said no, would he have assumed I could carry on in pain, so long as I could still be a productive member of society? Is a woman in pain not in enough pain until she can't work, until she can't take care of her children, until she's unable to be a satisfying sexual partner?

The other thing that happened when I tried to engage in a more masculine conversation about pain with a medical professional is that I used a lot more jargon. I worked in a hospital, and my medical terminology was pristine, probably better than most first-year medical students. I didn't necessarily put it on, but I didn't hesitate to use words that were highly specific, which I figured a doctor would appreciate. Doctors tend to dislike vagueness. It's kind of strange: when I enter into conversations with medical professionals outside of the office, they ask where I went to medical school. When I was in the office as a patient, however, I just got asked if I "Googled a lot" before coming in to the office. I was chastised in an "Aren't you cute?" kind of way that made me feel foolish.

The irony of being asked about medical school wasn't lost on me. I'd been out of college several years by then. If I'd never gotten sick—or if I had, at the very least, become well—I would have graduated in 2013. And in fact, I did go to commencement that year. As I watched Rebecca receive her diploma, it occurred to me that even if I did go back to Sarah Lawrence, I'd never be able to return to what it had been when I'd left. Not just because she and my other pals would no longer be there, but because I was not even the faintest remnant of the girl I'd been before.

When I left campus and came home, for the third and final time, I suppose I felt some closure. At the very least, I knew that I could only go in one direction: there was nothing that would change history. Short of some profound advancement in quantum physics, I would never be able to go back in time, only forward.

It might seem counterintuitive, but the first decision I made was to just not go to a doctor at all for the next year or so. I wasn't even trying to make a statement. I was just too tired, too broke, and had started to feel like I was living in that oft-cited definition of insanity: doing the same thing over and over again and expecting a different result. So instead, I got copies of my entire medical record, from every single hospital I'd ever been treated in, and I got to work.

If no one in my life, or anywhere else, for that matter, seemed to know much about endometriosis, I'd learn. And then, I'd teach them.

———✦———

I GREW UP STRADDLING TWO lives: one online and one offline. The teens I know today seem to have just one life that exists simultaneously in both universes, but for my generation it was a little clunkier. We spent the first half of our childhood without our own computers, and the latter half with groaning dial-up desktops that gave us merely a taste of what was to come. Almost overnight we went through puberty and so did the Internet, all of us emerging on the other side having become more sure of our capabilities, if not confident in our purpose.

My first blog was a mouthy, first-person lament called cLiCk-AbLe CaTasTrOpHe, which existed from the time I was about thirteen years old, up until a few years ago when Xanga wiped old blogs. I didn't write much about what was happening at the time, but rather, looked ahead to the future. I talked about what I wanted, what I was reaching for. I didn't have an audience for these musings (that I know of, anyway). But it didn't matter, it wasn't about the audience. It was about screaming into the void.

Throughout my teen years I developed an online voice through instant messaging and the early days of social media. I carefully curated a Myspace page, and I changed my AOL Instant Messenger handle as though it were a digital mood ring. The Internet also provided me with the same kind of reassurance as the library, or a set of encyclopedias. Before Google, there was Ask Jeeves, and trust me: I asked Jeeves a lot of weird shit. There were so many esoteric questions for which I had not yet found answers in books, and the Internet provided me with new avenues for exploration.

After I got sick, the Internet became an invaluable research tool—and a conduit through which I could connect to others, to know that I wasn't alone. I hated to think that there were other women out there, awake in bed at odd hours of the night, staring at their computer screens with the same kind of desperate, validation-seeking gaze I wore—but at the same time, I was terrified to think that I was experiencing something that was without precedent. I didn't want to be a pioneer in illness.

I wrote, I read, I listened—and I began to realize that the patients I'd been connecting with online shared many of the same fears. The same story repeated itself over and over and over again: my doctor didn't believe my pain was real, I can no longer have sex, I'm nauseated all the time and I can't eat, I'm so bloated I look five months pregnant, I'm so exhausted all the time I'm losing my ability to work, I'm terrified I'll lose my job, my husband, my children . . .

Many of these women were on forums reporting their symptoms, their experiences, without having the anchor of a diagnosis.

These women were from all backgrounds, all races, all ages. Some had mothers or sisters or aunts with endometriosis, or uterine cancer, or ovarian cancer. Some worried that they had cancer. Some worried that endometriosis might lead to cancer. Many worried they would never get pregnant. Some had managed to get pregnant only to have their symptoms return with a vengeance once their pregnancies ended. Many were no longer able to enjoy sex, but were having it anyway because they were afraid of losing their partners. Of losing themselves. Many had either lost their jobs, and been forced to go on disability, or were dangerously close to doing so. Almost all said that they felt alone, that no one in their lives really understood how they felt, because they didn't look sick most of the time.

Endometriosis is sometimes called an invisible illness, as a person may look fine on the outside, with no obvious sign that she is ill. It's an interesting characterization, but there is another meaning as well: sometimes endometriosis lesions are clear, and are thus even invisible to a surgeon staring directly at them. The lesions may be detectable only through tissue biopsy, which may or may not be performed, depending on the surgeon's level of knowledge.

It's true that those suffering from endometriosis haven't lost all their hair from chemotherapy or taken on that gray hue of a person with a terminal illness. They are not wheelchair bound or using a cane. They may well get up every day, wash their hair, put on makeup, get dressed, and go to work.

But they do suffer, likely far more than even those closest to them know. Especially in the moments when they are alone and can let their guard down. For me, it was usually in my car that I felt safe to fall apart, where I hid away to nap or fend off a bad wave of nausea. I'm sure everyone has their own place to escape to, or to sequester themselves where they can suffer privately. Lonely places that swallow the sounds, smells, and sights of pain, sucking the proof right out of the marrow, washing it away so that not even a filmy residue remains.

It would be noble of me to say that I started writing about my experiences because I wanted to reach out and help, but that impetus came later. At the beginning, I was writing purely as a means to understand my own grief. When I started yelling into the void of the Internet, I was startled when it began to whisper back.

Other women like me were out there, dying to be heard. After spending a few months digging through and considering what was in my own medical history, I put out a simple call on Twitter: if you have endometriosis, please answer these questions. I specifically encouraged people of color and LGBTQ folks to participate, as I was aware that their perspectives were woefully underrepresented. I attached a link to a Typeform I'd set up, which allowed people to answer the questions, include some demographic information and contact info, and choose whether they wanted to remain anonymous.

I received a small number of responses over the next week and was amazed at how varied they were. A few people I already knew—I had met them on the Internet through our mutual endo struggles—responded—but even more strangers answered. As I read through the responses and began to put together the larger picture of what life with endo is like for those of us who live with it, I found myself with more questions than answers.

I also started talking about endometriosis more openly offline, and when I brought it up, I found that I got one of two responses: "What's that?" or, "Oh, my [mother, sister, second cousin twice removed] has that!" The latter came a lot more frequently than I had expected. I noticed that it was often said dismissively, like, "Yeah, my sister's a brunette, too." At first I didn't challenge it or offer up anything else, for fear that I was going to overshare. But eventually my curiosity got the best of me.

Did people not realize how debilitating this condition was? That's a given, for those who don't know someone with it, and of course their ignorance is obvious, maybe even slightly forgivable. But for those who knew someone with endo, I couldn't believe how blasé they were about the whole thing. So I started asking more questions, risking sounding like I was entitled to other people's business. People often just shrugged, saying stuff like, "Well, she had trouble getting pregnant," and didn't seem to know much else. I'm sure if I'd pressed further, asked them to describe their family member's or friend's health, they would have shrugged and said, "Fine."

I had a sneaking suspicion that if I were to actually talk to the women in question, rather than talking about them, their version of endometriosis would probably be quite different. And the word "fine" probably wouldn't factor in—unless it was said through gritted teeth.

After the *Huffington Post* picked up a piece I wrote about endometriosis, women started emailing me or reaching out to me on Facebook to share their stories, or to tell me that I'd given them a voice.
They'd taken my article with them to their doctors, or shown it to their
spouses. They felt validated. I've lost count of the women who have
emailed me to say, "Thank you for making me feel like I'm not crazy."

Although these emails were gutting and overwhelming, they so
closely mirrored my own experience that I couldn't help but feel val-
idation myself. I hated thinking that so many women were suffering
the way I was—but what were the odds we were all just "making it
up"? There's strength in numbers, right?

IN THE FALL OF 2015, five years after the life-altering shower, I gave
a presentation at a medical conference at Stanford University. Stanford Medicine X is designed to make patients equal stakeholders with
physicians and researchers—no small task when you consider the hierarchy that dictates the health-care system in our country. I'd heard
about it on Twitter and submitted a presentation for consideration earlier in the year. It wove my personal narrative with that of others, and
explained the process by which I became an advocate for myself as
I journeyed through the US health-care system. My perspective was
unique, because at that point in time, I had been working *in* health
care for several years and was well acquainted with the system's dys-
functions and idiosyncrasies. I also believed that the hierarchy in
which it operated had long ago ceased to work, and was more than
happy to challenge its integrity. Mostly, though, I was looking forward to connecting with other patients with chronic illnesses who
had largely diagnosed themselves and devised innovative and practical ways to deal with their day-to-day needs.

Many of the patients at Stanford Medicine X were medical "zebras" with rare conditions, or diseases for which there is no known
cure. They are pioneers not just in their own care, but in the care
of anyone else with their condition. These patients are extraordinary
individuals who, instead of letting their disease strip their lives of
meaning, have forced it to give them a sense of purpose. They are
advocates, luminaries, researchers, teachers, brilliant and passionate

speakers—and above all, they are people who have been empowered by the fragility of life. Being among them, sharing my experience, made me consider that maybe I had not experienced a total loss in being ill, but instead, just a seismic shift in priorities.

When I finished my presentation, a physician approached me with a rather grave expression on his face. It took him a moment to gather himself, to get out what he wanted to say.

He looked at me quite intently, and at first I thought maybe he was going to ream me out because I had his profession. But as I watched him, I realized he was actually somewhat teary-eyed. He wasn't angry, he was moved.

"I can't stop thinking about how many patients like you I've sent home," he said, shaking his head. "How many patients I might've done this to."

Before I departed health care entirely, I left the medical records department and took a temporary job that would allow me to put my health literacy and patient advocacy experience to good use. The program was based out of the hospital system at large, not specifically the hospital I'd been working in, so early on in that process I was given the grand tour of the primary hospital's campus. Part of a larger group of new hires, I was walked through a literal Hall of Fame that was lined with photos: one for every CEO the hospital system had had since its inception. Although the photographs became of increasingly higher quality, and evolved from black and white to technicolor as we made our way through the decades, there was one very noticeable constant: they were all men. I knew this wasn't true at every level: I'd sat on committees myself, and taken notes for my boss in more than a few midlevel meetings over the years, so I knew that there *were* women in leadership roles—but only up to a certain point. I was more familiar with the administrative power structure in health care than the clinical one, but in casual conversation with physicians and nurses over the years I'd certainly gleaned that there was, undeniably, a "boys' club." No girls allowed.

INEXPLICABLE COINCIDENCES, CONNECTIONS, and an overdosing of pure luck has described my life thus far. I'm not sure if the connections are abundant or if I'm just unusually good at seeing them, but those breaths of splendid fortuity have saved my life on more than one occasion. Certainly they are always welcome, always enchanting.

I met Lorraine on the Internet because we both were part of an online group that faithfully watched *Downton Abbey* together each week and then thoroughly critiqued it. I actually wrote the weekly recaps for *The Mary Sue* during the last season, which bolstered my freelance writing career and legitimized my Tumblr rants. Lorraine, a fire-haired, twenty-something nurse from New Jersey, is a magnificent cosplayer. Her legendary collection of hand-sewn costumes, wigs, accessories, and props is astounding to my untrained eye, and I marvel at her many handicraft skills.

Although I had talked to Lorraine and the others in the group every week for a year, we'd never met in real life. I was preparing to take a trip to New York City to visit Rebecca, who had been living in Brooklyn since graduating from Sarah Lawrence. Lorraine lived in New Jersey, so it would be easy to meet up. She mentioned that she could come into the city with her father, who worked at Weill Cornell Medical College in Manhattan. We could meet for lunch, and since I had worked in health care and understood medicine well enough to appreciate its many exciting applications, she could show me around her father's office at the Skills Acquisition and Innovation Laboratory.

Lorraine looked exactly like she did in her online pictures, which I thought was hilarious, because oftentimes, that's not the case. We hugged, immediately fangirled over each other as her father procured some bagels, then carried on along Sixty-Eighth Street toward First Avenue, where we'd spend the better part of the day at Weill Cornell. When I had a chance to chat with her father, Dr. Rosenberg, and thank him for allowing me to visit the skills lab (which I was spellbound by), he asked me about myself and I explained the situation regarding my diagnostic odyssey and the research I was doing.

As soon as I mentioned my study was on endometriosis, he beamed. The universe had somehow handed me Lorraine, who led me to Dr. Rosenberg, who just so happened to be best friends with Dr. Harry Reich.

"Oh, Uncle Harry!" Lorraine laughed, "Yeah, he'd be a great interview."

My jaw nearly hit the floor. Dr. Reich was a world-renowned pioneer in laparoscopic surgery. He was also heavily involved with the Endometriosis Foundation of America (EFA), which I knew was an invaluable resource and had been eager to learn more about. Dr. Reich was certainly positioned high on the list of people I'd want to discuss endometriosis with.

"Here's his email," Dr. Rosenberg said, dropping his fountain pen back into the pocket of his white coat before leaving Lorraine and me to head off for lunch and a trip to Lush—the environmentally conscious bath bomb emporium you could smell from a mile away. "Tell him you're friends with my daughter."

So that's exactly what I did. As soon as I got back to Rebecca's apartment in Brooklyn that afternoon, I plopped down on her couch and crafted an email. Dr. Reich emailed me back almost immediately, saying simply, "Call me." He included his phone number. I never expect people to just hand out their phone numbers anymore. I mean, talking on the phone seems like a strictly personal activity to me, or a desperate matter of debt negotiation. I have an eternally dwindling list of people that I actually talk to on the phone, and the ones who remain are people with whom I am very intimate and comfortable. The only other time I use the phone is to call a credit card company or schedule a dentist appointment, and I usually have a few hours' worth of anxiety preceding the event.

Since I was calling Dr. Reich the same afternoon I'd emailed him, there hadn't been enough time for any apprehensiveness to fester, so I was fairly calm and collected. Besides that, given Dr. Reich's state of renown, I naturally assumed he'd think me a peon compared to the people he normally spoke to. So when he answered the phone and starting telling me, with a rather easy and casual tone, all about his connections to Maine, and his current level of stress related to helping plan the EFA's next conference (which was less than a month away), I was pleasantly surprised and quite relieved. He was extremely personable, and naturally wanted to know where in Maine I was from. He was currently visiting his grandchildren, he explained, and every few minutes I'd hear a child squealing or a dog barking, or he'd turn the receiver away from his mouth for a second to say something to someone. He told me he was recovering from surgery, chatting me up like we were old pals. Then, he volleyed me a most unexpected question: Would I like to speak at the conference as a patient?

I didn't hesitate to say yes—mostly because he'd also prefaced the offer by telling me about the vacancy he still had to fill for the conference's slate of speakers. But I also figured that accepting his offer would be even better than my original plan, which had been simply to attend as an observer, a writer, and a patient who was forever trying to unravel the mysteries of this disease. Here was one of the experts asking me to be a part of it at a much higher level, and from there, the view would no doubt be far more interesting.

⸺🙊

WHEN I RETURNED TO NEW York City a few weeks later to attend the conference, I was in the middle of a pretty bad flare-up of endo symptoms, which seemed fitting. The first day was Patient Day, where the physicians came together with patients and other people who were not necessarily interested in the academic part of the conference, but still wanted to learn about endometriosis. They could come hear some patient stories and learn about research efforts. I was to speak in the afternoon, which seemed impossibly far away, considering that within the first hour of being there, I'd soaked through three or four pads and taken two anti-nausea pills.

The presentations weren't that revealing to me, and I'm sure they weren't to many of the other patients in the room, either: we hear the same story over and over again from one another, hear ourselves telling it again and again to doctors, friends, lovers, bosses—this inescapable narrative having become something that none of us wants to be a part of, but at the same time, the very proof that we are not concocting some elaborate lie about the inner failings of our bodies. We are forced to seek out the suffering of others to validate our own.

Besides, the whole morning was really geared more toward doctors. I don't think it was intentional—but when medical professionals give speeches, they give speeches. By this time, I had a not insubstantial medical background, so I followed most of what they were saying, but I wondered how those in the room who did not understand felt. There were women in the room who, like me, probably understood but could not follow or make sense of the jargon, because they were exhausted, and in pain, and their intellects had no room to open up and bloom under the weight of their suffering.

The moment of revelation happened, for me, not during the speeches, but at a very specific moment during the first coffee break, when a large group of women tried to cram into a very small, two-stalled bathroom. I'm an observer by nature: had I not channeled my observations into writing, I would have liked to become an anthropologist. That bathroom was the purest, most unfettered kind of vignette that could have been in someone's case study on endometriosis. There we were, leaning against the cool tile of the bathroom wall or trying to suck in the fresh April air by crowding before the smallest of cracked windows next to the sink. We groaned and gritted our teeth, the pain we'd been sitting with finally more than we could bite down on, the nausea burning our stomachs, fatigue glazing over our eyes so that we had to remember to knit our brows together (so we'd look interested and not exhausted).

I glanced over at the trash can and felt a strange exhilaration run through me. There, atop the wads of damp paper towel, were several wrappers for those stick-on heating pads. The very ones I had in my hand that I was going to wrap around my pelvis and lower back. There were women bent over the sink, caught in a wave of nausea or an unrelenting cramp. Women with sallow, tear-stained cheeks who had no doubt come in here to cry. When I finally got into a stall, my legs were shaking as I tried to lower my body onto the toilet seat. The bin for sanitary napkins next to me was practically overflowing, and that familiar scent of hot metal hung in the air.

I realized that the talk I had planned to give wasn't the talk I needed to give. As I stumbled out of the bathroom back to my seat, I started mentally making cuts. I would say most of what I had set out to say, but I was no longer interested in talking to the doctors in the room. I would talk to the women.

I don't remember giving my brief speech, because I was in pain, and nauseated—but I know I spoke to the patients. Specifically, I spoke about an online community I'd started called Ask Me About My Uterus. We curated essays about everything from menstruation and miscarriage to menopause. We'd amassed a readership of around 10,000, which had confirmed my suspicion that people—not just women—wanted a space in which to have these conversations. Preferably in the world, with each other. But until then, online mediums would have to do.

While I allowed the essays to speak for themselves in terms of storytelling, I wanted to find a way to quantify the experiences that were being shared. Since I was going through all the submissions and had been, for quite some time, reading emails from women all over the world who would regularly send me their stories, I began to notice certain patterns. The only objective data I could offer up was what I could cull from their subjective experiences: What were the most common words used to describe these experiences? As the vast majority of those who had contributed were women, I was going back to my previous questions about how women talk about their pain. I tallied up the most frequently used words across all the essays that had been submitted to date, created a visual representation, and put it up before the audience for consideration. Of the top three words, the first two anyone could have guessed: pain and doctor. It was the third that had gripped me, and, I found, the people in the room before me: *time*.

At the end of that session, when the speakers all sat up at the front in a panel to take questions, no one asked me any questions. But afterward, when the day was over and I was trying to navigate my way out of the building, women began coming up to me in tears. They were thankful that someone had spoken to them, about them.

Dr. Reich, still using a cane after a recent knee surgery, limped over to introduce me to his wife and a few other physicians. They included Dr. Tamer Seckin, who founded the Endometriosis Foundation of America with Padma Lakshmi. When Lakshmi was in her thirties, Dr. Seckin was the first doctor to take her symptoms seriously. Together, they formed the EFA to help raise awareness. Along with the annual medical conference, each year they throw a gala event that helps raise money—the Blossom Ball. The 2016 speakers included Padma, Lena Dunham, and Susan Sarandon—all three of whom have endometriosis. Although I'd been able to attend the duration of the medical conference, I couldn't afford a ticket to the gala event. When someone mentioned they needed volunteers to check people in and take tickets, I volunteered. I had to borrow a little black dress from Rebecca. (The one dress I'd brought with me had fit me the week before when I'd packed it, but my endo symptoms made everything about it—from its cut to the fabric—insufferable.)

The medical conference lasted a couple of days, and although I took copious notes for later reviewing, I was in so much pain that I wondered at the end of each day if I'd wake up well enough for the next. Irony circled me as I sat there, downing my pills with catered coffee. I listened to some of the world's best medical minds explain their pioneering, life-altering research about endo. I watched man after man after middle-aged man step up to the podium and proclaim that he could cure endometriosis—with a sense of bravado that made me squirm. I flipped through the program and saw my name under the conference faculty list, since I'd spoken at Patient Day, and realized I was the only person on the list without an alphabet soup of degrees after their name. I suspected I might well have been the only person on that list who actually had endometriosis.

I suddenly felt ridiculous being there. My suffering hadn't given me any real power, not the kind of power you need to effect change. What I needed was the education that endo had ripped from me. When I'd spoken at Patient Day, I'd opened with what I felt was a necessary disclaimer, a self-effacing remark that was totally improvised, but that I felt was necessary since it was obvious I was there despite any kind of legitimate medical education, something I'm still very self-conscious about.

"Hi, I'm Abby Norman. I am not a doctor—but I might have been."

It kind of became my standard opener after that, but upon further reflection, I realized there may have been more than a grain of truth in it. When I got sick that September at Sarah Lawrence, a biology course was the last lecture I ever attended. It was aptly titled "The Biology of Living and Dying." By the time I left Sarah Lawrence I certainly was more concerned with the biology of dying than I'd been when I'd started. And oddly enough, there were some prescient hints in my chosen thesis topic for the year: I'd been interested in studying the phenomenon of apoptosis, programmed cell death. While cells often die as a result of necrosis, which causes tissue death, apoptosis is a more intentional kind of demise. It's sort of like controlled demolition. There are times when it makes sense, from a molecular biology standpoint, for a cell to orchestrate its own end, because it senses some kind of disturbance in the molecular field. Or, alternatively, it can be driven to do so by communications it receives from other cells. These intrinsic and extrinsic pathways were fairly under-researched until the early 1990s, but in the past twenty years, so-called cell suicide has become a fascination across multiple scientific disciplines.

I'd become interested with the topic after seeing the word "apoptosis" in a textbook. I had looked up its Greek origin and found that the word meant "falling off," as in the falling of leaves from the trees in autumn, which was perhaps my favorite thing in the world.

But I never progressed much beyond that, because within six weeks of sitting in the quad beneath a tree whose leaves were only beginning to think about making their final descent, I was back in Maine, motionless in bed, listening to the trees snapping outside my window, trees that were sending their leaves plummeting to the ground, indifferent to their consent.

But the trees were blossoming, white and pungent, on those little strips of grass along the median of the Upper West Side, as I sipped my coffee in a conference room at the Union Club—an interesting place to hold a conference that was concerned primarily with the nuances of the female reproductive system. It's one of New York City's oldest private men's-only social clubs, and historically a very conservative one. As I mulled over the irony of this, I looked up to see Dr. Seckin standing over me.

"We missed you at the faculty dinner last night," he said. I blinked, stuttering out a response that indicated I had not realized I was invited. He laughed at this, saying of course I'd been invited. Someone else caught his attention and he drifted back into the crowd, and I slumped down in my seat.

I had received a phone call a few days before but had completely forgotten about it, at least partially because I was feeling so ill. While they had been drinking sparkling wine and dining in some beautiful banquet hall, I was doubled over on the Q train trying to make it back to Brooklyn before I passed out.

I'd been hoping that if I managed to rest each evening after the conference, by the time the Blossom Ball came around I might actually feel halfway decent. I didn't, but I had promised to take tickets, so I showed up. I wore Rebecca's black dress—in fact, I'd been wearing it all day. It was simple and elegant but a little underwhelming for the occasion, which turned out to be filled with Hollywood glamour.

I was nervous about volunteering, not because the people were famous, but because I felt like shit and looked even worse. They'd probably come down the hall and take one look at me and think they were in the wrong place. As it turned out, the opposite happened—and people seemed to be lining up in front of me to be checked in, somewhat inexplicably. The other volunteers laughed about it, and I couldn't seem to find any rationale—but then I realized that it was actually quite simple: I was wearing my glasses. I'd vowed not to (as I'm constantly told they spoil my looks), but I couldn't see the iPad in front of me without them. As one of the other volunteers pointed out, amid the glitz and glamour of the city's most rich and famous, my unassuming and completely genuine dowdiness probably put people at ease.

I had never seen such opulence before, though I figured out pretty quickly that most famous people (and their many, many handlers) are just as exhausted by the minutiae of public appearances or events as "regular" people would be. I specifically remember watching Allison Williams fix her hair in front of a mirror in the hallway before she hit the red carpet where all the photographers had squished themselves in; they proceeded to yell incessantly from every direction, issuing commands like "Over the shoulder!" and "All the way to the right!" She seemed resigned to it all, but I grew weary watching her. I just wanted to give her a snack.

As the night wore on, I found a spot on the back wall where I could lean and watch people, although I failed to notice that my position, paired with my entirely black wardrobe, made me look like a member of the catering team. After being asked for crudités one too many times, I grabbed a glass of wine from the bar, straightened my back, and worked the room—albeit reluctantly.

The room was full of interesting people, many of whom I had already met or had seen on television, so why was I hiding away in the corner? My attempts to bolster my energy were futile. I was just tired.

It was getting late and I felt wildly irrelevant. I was slightly re-juvenated when I spotted Dr. Reich and his wife across the room. When I went to say hi, he invited me to sit down at his table—I pro-tested, because tables had been reserved for the Guggenheims and other people who would donate money, and all I had in my purse was my Metrocard and a debit card that had a wad of gum stuck to it. I hadn't been able to find a trash can earlier, as the gala was being held at one of those event centers that had trash cans that didn't look like trash cans, and decorative ornaments that did look like trash cans but were not. So I'd just stuck my gum in my purse.

I chatted with Dr. Reich's wife and their son. I had a glass of wine. Suddenly people were interested in me, in my writing. All the doctors were interested in my experience with endo. They were alarmed, miffed, when I admitted I was still suffering. In fact, right before them in that moment, I was in pain. Several of them said dif-ferent versions of the same thing: "Why not come to me? I'll fix you."

And my answer was always the same: "I can't afford to see you." Hell, if I hadn't volunteered, I wouldn't have even been able to afford to buy a ticket to the gala. I couldn't even afford to be standing there. I definitely couldn't afford the Cabernet Sauvignon.

At the end of the evening, I shook Padma Lakshmi's hand and wondered if she was tired. I bid farewell to Dr. Reich, thanked him profusely for his help with my research, for taking me to lunch the day before, for being genuinely approachable. Then, I stood out on the curb in front of Pier 60, waiting for the Uber that Rebecca and her roommate had called for me, since I was too exhausted to take the subway all the way back to Brooklyn in the middle of the night.

A group of people appeared next to me, a tall, sparkling woman in the middle of them. They were laughing, loudly joking around the way my friends and I used to in high school. A large black SUV pulled up, with its blacked-out windows, and I realized it was Padma and her entourage. I watched them pile into this car, my last vision of her just a foot in a strappy heel disappearing into the night.

I chuckled. I bet she couldn't wait to get out of those goddamn shoes.

CHAPTER 8

Nothing happens in contradiction to nature, only in
contradiction to what we know of it. And that's a
place to start. That's where the hope is.

—Dana Scully, *The X-Files*

AS THE INTERNET WIDENED MY world and allowed me to connect with the experiences of people across time and distance, I realized that where I wasn't having these conversations was in my real life. Perhaps the text-based communication of the Web, and the distance afforded by cyberspace, made it easier for people to be forthcoming.

So, when I got a message from a friend I hadn't spoken to in years saying that she was getting ready to have a hysterectomy and wanted to talk to me about it, I was quite excited. I tried not to be too eager, though. Stefanie was thirty-five years old. It occurred to me that if she was having a hysterectomy at that age, there was likely a serious reason—and it may not be one to celebrate.

When she bustled into the coffee shop in the small Midcoast Maine town we both called home, she didn't look distraught. Maybe a little frazzled, but she was the mother of two children under the age of five, one of whom—a baby girl—she and her husband had only adopted just before Christmas. Quite literally *just* before: they got "the call" three days before the holiday and then spent the first few weeks of the year out of state while the adoption paperwork was processed. Although I really only knew Stefanie peripherally, I did know this about her: she was the epitome of mom-material, and she'd be the first to tell you that. "Growing up we played with baby dolls, we practiced taking care of them, we practiced giving *birth* to them," she laughed, sipping out of a little cartoon-character-covered water bottle that probably belonged to one of her kids—but given her sweet nature could just as well have been hers. She caught me up on their daughter's adoption story, and the bittersweet weight of it was not lost on me. I remembered quite vividly when Stefanie had lost her first daughter, Rose.

The summer I'd met Max, I'd been in a community theater production of *Peter Pan*; Stefanie had been the Peter to my Wendy. My first impression of her, which endures, was that she was a remarkably delightful person. She's wide-eyed and excitable, and as a children's librarian and lover of Disney, she was clearly the perfect Pan both onstage and off. The kids in the cast adored her, and I'll never forget how she got me the cutest cupcake—topped with a marzipan acorn—on the final night of the run.

I'll also never forget being backstage, my brow knit with concern as she sat on the stairs before me looking a bit peaked, when she'd told me—in strictest confidence, but with an unmistakable gleam in her eye—that she was pregnant. As it turned out, she'd been trying for quite some time, but had suffered two previous miscarriages, from which she was still understandably traumatized.

In retelling the story to me now, years later, she began by saying that her periods had always been very intense. "I remember in high school writhing on the bathroom floor with cramps, vomiting, flushing hot, waiting for someone to take me home," she said. "Even on birth control in college and when I was first married, that second day would still be rough. I was diagnosed with PCOS [Polycystic Ovarian Syndrome], which made ovulating tricky and just getting pregnant very difficult. My cycles in between were beyond horrible."

After the miscarriages, her periods took on an entirely new power: as an emotional trigger. "The sight of so much blood, the intense cramps, and this horrible sliding feeling as huge clots came out of me was just like my miscarriages," she said. "I was immediately reliving all that crap again. When my own body is triggering the PTSD and the loop just keeps cycling through, it's overwhelming."

When she finally got pregnant a third time, she was cautiously optimistic. She knew the statistics about miscarriage—which were higher in her case, since she'd already had two. Her voice grew quieter and she added, "And 1 out of 160 pregnancies ends with a stillbirth."

She was twenty-seven weeks pregnant when she stopped feeling the baby kick. Something was wrong, and Stefanie knew it, but she didn't want to go to the hospital. She didn't want a doctor to tell her— *again*—that she'd lost the baby. Several hours later, when she finally heard the dreaded words, she thought the situation couldn't possibly get worse. Then, the doctor explained that she'd have to be admitted to deliver. This didn't compute at first—wouldn't she just miscarry the same way she had twice before? Then it hit her: she was too far along. What they meant was that she would have to give birth to her stillborn daughter.

Over the next three days, she was "pumped so full of Pitocin it blew out my vein." She delivered on November 21, 2011. "When the placenta wouldn't detach, a whole crew of people suddenly filled my room. Holding onto my legs, ultrasounding me, pulling." She did not get to hold her daughter for very long afterward, and was then sent to recover in the OB unit, where she could hear babies crying through the night. She asked the nurse for a fan to put in her room. "I left the hospital with a little purple memory box with her footprints, hospital bracelet, hat, and a few pictures. I had to call and arrange for an urn and flowers for a memorial," she recalled. "We only just installed a headstone in 2016 because it was too painful to even think about. Too final."

After two miscarriages and a stillbirth, there was a lot of asking *why*. They expected that it might take a bit of investigation, so they were prepared to wait. But the first specialist they saw immediately wanted to test Stefanie for an autoimmune condition called antiphospholipid antibody syndrome, which causes the blood to clot too much.

Stefanie was positive for it. No sooner had they suspected there was a mysterious force at work than it had been solved by a simple blood test. Stefanie had miscarried, and her daughter had been stillborn, because the veins in her uterus were clotting up and causing the placenta to fail.

When she got pregnant again she had to work very closely with her doctors and give herself twice-daily shots of anticoagulants. "What the doctor wasn't telling me as I was having all these tests and being monitored," Stefanie said, "was that he was waiting for my placenta to fail. Because it was going to."

Not wanting to alarm her about it, the doctor had simply kept a close enough eye on her that when the moment seemed imminent, he could admit her for an emergency Caesarean section. She was a month away from her due date—and having ultrasounds every seventy-two hours—when it happened.

"I didn't have a car seat, I hadn't taken a birthing class, I didn't even have a change of clothes," she recalled. When her son, Liam, was born, he was tiny: 4 pounds, 12 ounces. He went immediately to the neonatal intensive care unit (NICU). Stefanie's husband was stricken. "He thought he was saying goodbye," she told me. But Liam, though small, was fierce. He wasn't in the NICU long, because he kept yanking off all his monitoring equipment. Today, he's doing well: he takes growth hormones, though he'll likely always be on the small side. His parents can't be sure exactly how his life will be affected by his condition—which they learned is called Russell-Silver syndrome.

Becoming a mother did not, of course, alleviate the grief Stefanie felt for the loss of her daughter, or mitigate the trauma of her previous miscarriages. "I miss Rose every day," she said. "But I've learned how to manage that, keep it dulled, and work through it in a healthy way." Her periods, which have continued to send her back into that space emotionally and physically, have become a cruel and seemingly inescapable trigger. "But when that physical sensation of my cycle is happening, I can't get away from reliving it. I feel the bathroom tile on my face during the second miscarriage. I feel hands pulling at me to get the placenta out. I cry because I didn't get to hold Rosie long enough after. I can feel the wind on my face as my husband and I lower her urn into the ground. And it's all replayed with such awful, vivid clarity."

I understand, then, why she wanted to talk to me. To process her decision—or, really, her realization—that a hysterectomy was a choice she could make. "My stupid reproductive system, which has caused all the problems in the first place, is now exacerbating the situation. So, I decided it needs to go." She looks relieved just thinking about it; her entire demeanor softens, relaxes. She points out that although a doctor wouldn't have consented to an elective hysterectomy on the basis of her trauma alone, her blood disorder is more than enough to qualify it as medically necessary. Quite simply, she can't safely be on hormonal birth control because of her high risk for blood clots. Regardless of how the procedure needed to be framed to satisfy the medical profession or the insurance company, the outcome would be the same: freedom.

"In June they are going to scoop that sucker out and I can finally not be forced to have my own body turned against me," she said.

Throughout history, medical science has been convinced of the womb's potential to make a woman ill—to the extent that hysterectomies (consented to or not) were an accepted treatment. Whether the reasons were purely medical or, often, partly psychiatric is debatable. But it was the physician's assessment, not the woman's experience, that determined whether her uterus was the culprit. A physician's interpretation of a woman's pain and suffering, of her stability or instability, was what led to treatment.

Stefanie's uterus had become a source of both physical pain and emotional anguish. Empowered through her experiences, she was turning hundreds of years of hysteria on its head. She was reclaiming her body, her life, her *self*.

THE WORD "PAIN" COMES FROM the Latin *poena*, meaning "punishment or penalty," and for many women like Stefanie—or like me—that is at times precisely what it feels like. When I became darkly depressed and wanted to kill myself, the doctors gave me medication that made me feel like a damp washcloth. I ran the gamut of emotions from uppercase A to lowercase a. I didn't feel good—I just no longer felt the need to get up at 2 a.m. and Google how to suffocate myself with a shopping bag. I was still in pain, I still felt sick, but I no longer expected that my life would, or should, be any different. Depression, and the numbness afforded to me by way of an antidepressant, made me feel like my lot in life was to suffer. I stopped expecting my life to get better. So it didn't.

I was unusually concerned with justice when I was a little girl. The kids on the playground hated me because I was definitely a rat. If I witnessed someone breaking rules, I tattled. But I also held myself to that standard. When I did something wrong, I likewise held myself accountable, sometimes to the extreme. I was just as likely to tattle on myself as I was someone else, because I wanted to believe that the world was a just place. Then I grew up and realized the world beyond recess was corrupt, and that sometimes good people got shot in the street for no reason, and bad people became high-ranking government officials with salaries and boats named after beautiful women. Life was not particularly fair—but that didn't mean everything was a punishment.

Still, part of me felt like I was sick because I had been happier than I deserved to be. Up until I went to Sarah Lawrence, I had lived in a permanent state of fight-or-flight. I hadn't known where I'd be sleeping from week to week, what I'd eat or when, whom to trust, who would hurt me or who might help. Then, I had this magical period of rest for eighteen months, and it came to a sudden, horrifying, literally gut-wrenching end. The loss of that taste of life was something I've struggled to grieve; admitting that I will never have it again is to admit that I will never be the person I was before I got sick. That my life was forever altered in a way that I could not control.

Endometriosis has always been indifferent to everything that has happened in my life. It may or may not have been there when I was hiding in the closet listening to the washing machine, before my ovaries even knew what to do with themselves. Some doctors, like Dr. Reich, believe that endometriosis is present at birth and becomes problematic once menstruation begins, sometimes crescendoing with ruptured cysts, or torqued tubes, or infections—like mine did. Some doctors believe other things, but to my knowledge, no doctor has posed a theory that endometriosis is a punishment for little girls who were bad, who left their families and tried to have a better life. Neither is cancer a punishment, or mental illness, or a really bad case of the flu.

I do think that the things that have happened to us in our lives inform how we confront illness, however. And many an anthropologist would agree: how we cope with everything from the inconvenience of a cold to a diagnosis that will change our lives says a lot not only about who we are, but about what illness represents to us. That representation doesn't just come from our parents, but from our lineage. From the society in which we live. Across time and space and culture, though, the feeling of being ill—particularly if it's sudden—makes us question what it means to be in control of our bodies. Of our lives. Of ourselves.

When I was a teenager and an expert in psychology and metaphysics (as all teenagers are), I thought I was someone who saw a loss of control as an opportunity to change direction. Given the things that happened to me during those years and the quick succession with which they did, I suppose I never had much of a choice. But when I got sick, I fought it. Looking back at journal entries, at emails sent to friends, at Facebook posts—I hadn't felt "right" for weeks, if not months, but I hadn't listened to my body because I didn't want to hear it. I was angry and afraid that I would lose everything. Then, after I confronted the reality of losing it all, I was angry and afraid that I would never get it back.

Then, I never got it back. And I had two choices: I could either stay bitter and disappointed about what I didn't have, what I would never have, or I could see the loss of control as an opportunity to change direction again. The hurdle was, I didn't want to go in any direction other than the one I'd been going in when I got sick. But that road was a dead end.

For awhile, I dug myself a hole and became very intimately aware of my own grief. I thought if I sat down there for long enough, alone in the musty darkness, that someone would toss me a rope and pull me out. But no one did. And one day, a little bit of light found its way in there. It warmed a corner of my face. The next day, a little more sun, a little more warmth.

Eventually, I popped my head up and looked around. Life had gone on without me. Trees had grown, flowers had sprung up, rabbits were happily copulating at an alarming rate. Frank Ocean finally put out a new album.

For awhile I merely watched. But at least I had started to look forward to sticking my head out and watching the world go by. In my world of pain, I slowly became aware of the life all around me. It served as a nice distraction. Sometimes I'd stick an arm out and wave someone over. Sometimes I'd reach out and feel the Earth, tug at the grass. Then, one day, I stood up. And I realized that the hole itself had never been what was keeping me in it—it had been my reluctance to stand up.

Getting out of the hole and back into the world didn't change the fact that I felt sick and was in pain, but I no longer felt quite so alone. The first thing I did was get a dog—Whimsy. Having responsibility for a dog, of course, meant I had to leave the house every day—even if only to take her for a short walk. Even on the days when that was nearly impossible, she was patient as I inched down the driveway. She's a rescue dog with a lot of emotional problems. We're an ideal match.

I stopped fighting my afternoon nap requirement. I tried to find things that my stomach could tolerate that were also nutritious. I drank more tea and went to bed by 9 p.m. every night. I finally decided that I could either try to live my life the way I'd wanted to, where I would continuously fail because I was asking too much of my body, or I could design an entirely new life. I admit, thinking about the prospect made me tired, but I decided it would be an ongoing process. I didn't have to plan it all out at once. I would get up each day and try, adding in the stuff that worked and letting go of what didn't.

Sometimes this meant people. Sometimes it meant expectations, or some kind of food. Whenever I lost something, I tried to imagine another space opening up inside of me that could be the place where something new would be seeded to grow. And who was I to say that it might not be something spectacular? My body was, after all, clearly skilled at taking me by surprise.

Even as I proselytized this new way of living to myself, there were still times when I needed to be sad or get angry about my situation. Especially when it meant having to say no to something I would much rather have said yes to. There were certainly days when I found the entire thing perfectly unreasonable, unfair, and bastardly.

One day, in the middle of a particularly frown-worthy bath, I remembered something that Jane had said to me years ago, back when I first got sick and would lay pitifully on the couch in her office. I was raw with disappointment that I wouldn't be able to go back to Sarah Lawrence, that I probably wouldn't graduate from college at all, that I'd never be the woman I wanted to be, or have the life I'd promised myself in order to get through all those difficult years.

"I just want to have a normal life," I said, wiping my tears on my sleeve. She didn't say anything at first, so I looked over at her. She was kind of curling her mouth around a smile. Then she sighed, raising her eyebrows knowingly at me.

"What about your life up until this point has made you think that it would ever be normal—?"

I'd sulked, of course, not daring to admit she might be onto something. Then she'd continued on with one of her "Your job is to take care of yourself" speeches. Only this time, when she realized I wasn't buying a word of it, she paused, waiting for me to look up.

"You can do it," she said softly, her eyes sincere. "You've done some magnificent things." At this, the tone of her voice seemed lilting, as if to add, *and you will do more of them.*

At the time, the sentiment fell flat for me because most days the most magnificent thing I aspired to was climbing a flight of stairs without having to stop at the top to rest. As my life carried on, carrying me with it, the idea that I could live a reasonably decent life even if I felt miserable seemed a better prospect than feeling miserable and living a miserable life.

I regained that anticipatory magic I'd had as a dancer. If I listened to my body, I knew what it wanted, what it needed, and I could heed the warnings. Sometimes I didn't end up feeling nearly so bad as I would have, had I tried to ignore it. I stopped expecting myself to make huge plans in advance, so that I wouldn't have to live in worry of not being able to keep them. I no longer attempted to eat food I knew would make me sick for the sole purpose of keeping up appearances, or out of fear of being rude. If I was in pain, and people asked how I was, I didn't lie. Some days I felt all right, and some days I didn't, but I stopped lying to people about it. Most importantly, I stopped lying to myself about it.

AFTER LIVING MY LOW-IMPACT, truth-telling, reasonable life for about six months, things were going pretty well. I was earning money. I was walking my dog. I visited with friends. I read books. I was writing a book, actually. This book. Or a collection of Nordic erotica—you'll never know for sure. Then, one morning I woke up, got out of bed, and realized my entire left side was numb.

Endometriosis has, at times, given me the sensation of sciatica in one of my legs. Usually my right leg, which is of course "my driving leg." At times it's been so painful that I can't drive, and it goes right from my sacrum down my butt and then down the back of my thigh like a buzzing electrical current. The sensation I woke up with wasn't quite that, but I was willing to believe it was related. Anytime over the years that I'd had some kind of lower-body symptom—pain, weakness—I'd assumed it was because I had endo too close to a nerve. In fact, I've known a lot of women to complain about sciatic pain during their periods.

Despite my new attitude about life, the preceding six months had been challenging health-wise. Over the winter, I'd actually gotten shingles, which was bizarre because of my age. Shingles usually hits people in the fifty-and-older set, unless you have a seriously compromised immune system. Which, of course, my doctors reasoned I did. I would tell you more about shingles, but I don't remember much about the ten days I was in bed. I was not particularly conscious. I was in excruciating nerve pain. Shingles is caused by the same herpes virus that causes chicken pox. Once you've had chicken pox, the virus stays in your nerve receptors forever, except it stays dormant, not bugging you in any way unless for some reason it gets reactivated. Shingles lesions erupt along a meridian of nerves and cause sores on your skin, usually your torso. Some people get them on their face. They burn like the fires of hell. Having that kind of nerve pain put into perspective to me just how vast the experience of pain really is. It was unlike any pain I'd experienced before, consuming in its heat. It was also fascinating, because it was not like the pain I had been living with daily for five years. In fact, while I had shingles, I was so overwhelmed with that sensation that I couldn't perceive the pain of my endo as clearly.

I have a brief memory of being too weak to hike up my shirt in the doctor's office, so the nurse practitioner had to help. I didn't even care that she was looking at my tits straight on. The shingles lesions went from my spine around the left side of my back and then to the front of my chest—right across my boob. For ten days I fantasized about cutting my own nipple off, because it probably would have been less painful. I'd already injured that breast once, as a very small child. I'd fallen onto the sharp end of some kind of push-toy, which lanced me right under the nipple. It bled for hours, and finally my parents took me to the emergency room, only to be told that the doctor could put a stitch in it, but that might mean I'd grow up with one normal boob and one Frankenboob. I guess the bleeding eventually slowed down because they didn't stitch me up. I still have the scar.

The shingles lesions healed within a few more weeks, but I remained rundown. In the spring, after being somewhat nudged by the Endometriosis Foundation conference, I went back to Dr. Paulson to ask if another laparoscopy might be warranted. I felt ready to do something more definitive, if necessary. Whether that meant she would have to refer me to someone else, or she herself yanked out an ovary, I didn't care. I was beginning to feel desperate, and a little embarrassed. As though I'd gotten lazy and hadn't been advocating hard enough to get better care. Of course, that's a lofty task when you're poor and sick all the time.

She reviewed my blood work and my physical exam and announced that no, she wouldn't do the surgery, as she felt I was too sick to go under anesthesia. I felt quite trapped by that assessment, and somehow slightly responsible for it. What if I'd come six months earlier, before I got shingles? What if I hadn't talked myself into all that feel-good bullshit and had kept banging down doctors' doors? What if I hadn't traded those medical textbooks for contemporary fiction? Once again I felt that I'd made the wrong choice, that I'd fucked it all up. I certainly was feeling like I couldn't win no matter what I did.

And that was how it felt when I woke up one morning in late April 2016 and couldn't feel the left side my body. At first I was afraid I was having a stroke—I'd read something that said that after you get shingles, your stroke risk goes up temporarily. But then again, it was also possible that I'd slept funny—and the totem of medicine is that when you hear hooves, you should look for horses, not zebras. I gave the dog her breakfast and we went out for our walk, taking the stairs one at a time, because I wasn't feeling steady on my feet. As we made our way down the road, I kept dropping her leash. Walking became increasingly difficult. It felt like I was wearing heavy rain boots filled with sand, or trying to wade through a sea of molasses. I went back to bed, reasoning that I was run down from the trip to New York, that I was stressed out about writing a book, and that I needed a better pillow.

Then, I started to lose my mind. I would be speaking and not be able to find the words I wanted, something that had never happened to me before. I've always been very articulate, always been able to memorize things, my recall quick and accurate. I started saying words that were close to the words I wanted, but not quite the right ones, which was even more perplexing. I also found that I couldn't follow conversations easily—I would get stuck a few beats behind. That was very alarming to me; I had never experienced anything like it even when I had been at my worst level of physical fatigue. Through all of my struggles with endometriosis, my mind had been quick and clever. A friend once said of me, "She has a wit so sharp she needs a permit." It had been how I'd survived everything. It had been what helped me save my own life, because it drove me to pore over medical journals and sort through record after medical record.

I'd slowly been coming to terms with the limitations of my physical body. I'd accepted that I could no longer dance, have sex, or eat food that wasn't basically a slight variation on bland. I'd figured I'd be okay because I could still think, and plan, and dream. I have a vivid imagination and can weave stories. I can bring a narrative to life within my mind that can entertain me the way my own life, at times, can no longer.

The thought of losing my mind was too much, so I called my doctor. By the time I picked up the phone, it was probably weeks later than I should have called, but I was analyzing my symptom differentials as well as I could. Years and years of seeing medical records coming across my desk, primarily for people who were middle-aged and older, had given me a pretty good internal repository of information, especially for neurological symptoms and orthopedic complaints.

I reasoned that I probably hadn't had a stroke, because it had been a few weeks since my new symptoms had appeared and I hadn't died yet. Perhaps I'd developed some kind of peripheral neuropathy from the shingles, though I wondered why it would show up suddenly instead of coming on gradually. Then I wondered if it had come on gradually, but I hadn't noticed because I'd been slowly losing my mind. I couldn't remember what my labs had said when my gynecologist had deemed me "too sick for surgery," but I considered that my B12 might be low, giving me muscle problems and considerable brain farts. I knew my white blood cell count was low, but it had been low for five years, and had gotten a little lower every time I had blood drawn. Maybe that was a clue, but it could also conceivably be the result of having had several serious infections in the span of a few years. I also wasn't eating well, despite having anti-nausea medication, because I didn't want to have to take it every day, and therefore tried to withstand low-grade nausea most days, only taking it when it was truly severe. But nutritional deficiencies had plagued me my entire life, and this was the first time I'd experienced something like this.

Except, it wasn't. In going back through my medical records for this book, I'd remembered a terrible experience I'd had in the hospital when I was in high school, when they called my mother because they didn't believe I was emancipated. I'd been there to see a neurologist for leg weakness, not unlike what I was experiencing now. True, the neurological deficits were new, but maybe these two things were connected.

I added a few possibilities to my potential diagnosis: lupus, multiple sclerosis, chronic Lyme disease—which wouldn't have been unusual, given that I live in Maine where it's practically endemic. I realized as I looked at my list that I didn't really know anything about any of the conditions I'd written down. Not that I was an expert on endometriosis, but I was an expert in *my* endometriosis. And although I knew that many people with endo wind up having additional, concurrent autoimmune diseases, an autoimmune disease like lupus seemed like more than I felt prepared to contemplate, let alone accept.

So I went to my regular doctor's office. Over the years, Dr. Gish had always been sympathetic to my concerns, but she had simply been directing traffic—sending me hither and thither, because she was a general practitioner. Still, I liked her and trusted her to, at the very least, be kind to me. I never expected that much of other doctors. I also knew that Dr. Gish saw a lot of patients, many of whom probably had the conditions I'd listed in my differential, given the demographic of patients. If something was there to be seen, I trusted her to see it. Because now, oddly enough, my body finally looked sick, and it was misbehaving in a way that was far more obvious than endometriosis had ever been. Or, if endometriosis was the culprit, now I had proof that could refute the characterization of it being an invisible illness.

These thoughts ran through my head as she examined me, but I didn't share them. I was also telling myself that it was entirely possible that she'd say there was nothing seriously wrong—that it was a pinched nerve, and I did just need a new pillow. But when she conducted a brief neurological exam, I faltered. I realized that I wasn't acing it, and suddenly a panic came over me. I knew this panic; it was what I'd felt when I'd first gotten sick. What I'd felt those nights when I'd lain awake in my bed crying out in pain, when no one was there to hear me, knowing that there was something inside me that was infected, or sick, or shouldn't be there, and that it would kill me if I didn't figure out what it was. It was the kind of panic that grabs you and shakes you, screaming, "Shut up and listen to me!"

Dr. Gish made a note in my chart and I slunk down from the exam table back into a nearby chair. My mind tripped over what little I could remember about neurological disorders, about autoimmune diseases, about hysteria—even about endometriosis. Then I stopped. I stopped thinking and I listened. Static crackled in my left side, like the TVs of my childhood that wouldn't come in unless the antenna was angled just right. I thought of all the times I would sit quietly and try to see inside my body, try to imagine what was inside of me causing pain, twisting my organs and filling my pelvis with fluid and blood. I closed my eyes, listening to Dr. Gish typing, and imagined sitting on my ribcage, hanging on and dangling my feet over the edge, having a literal heart-to-heart with my heart. What are you trying to tell me? I'm listening, tell me. I opened my eyes. Dr. Gish looked up at me, a curious but not unkind expression on her face.

"You said you have a gut feeling. I'd like to know what it is," she said.

It was clear that she already had a theory. I'd regaled her with my symptoms—the seemingly forever ones, the new more abrupt and frightening ones. I could see in her eyes that she had something, a possibility that needed concrete appreciation before she'd be confident enough to plaster it on me.

And yet, she was still interested in how I felt. Dr. Gish, unlike many other doctors I'd seen over the years, regarded the work I'd done to become an expert in my own body as worthwhile. It was astounding, but—even after all the time that I'd passed on the diagnostic carousel—this was the first time a medical professional had asked me how I felt with a sense that my opinions had any legitimacy.

Whatever the answer was, as yet unknown, existed within me. Even the most brilliant physician, who can have his or her hands rummaging around in of me, can never fully understand how it feels to live in my body. At times, I struggle to articulate how it feels myself, but I continue to learn, and adapt, and try to make sense of it.

Had I not persisted, I most certainly would have gone years, if not decades, without knowing that I had endometriosis. Had I not brought up the possibility of chronic appendicitis and insisted on further investigation, I most certainly would have died when it ruptured or from subsequent sepsis.

Still, after all that I'd been through, there was one fundamental truth that was still intact: I had never wanted to be right; I had only wanted to be well. You would have thought that with each correct diagnosis I made I would have developed more confidence in my perception of my body, but I still got lost in the whirl of questioning. I was insecure about my success in figuring out what was making me sick, partly because in doing so, ultimately, I had to accept that I was.

The clock ticked in the exam room, seeming to hesitate so as not to drown out my response as it drove us forward in time. I knew what I would tell her, but I was afraid to hear the words aloud. If I said it, would it manifest? If I didn't, would it thrive in my silence? Something else besides fear sidled up to me in the exam room—a familiar feeling of hopelessness.

Dr. Gish waited patiently for my response, perhaps sensing how tired I was of doing this. It was not so much perfunctory hopelessness, merely exhaustion. Yet after everything I'd been through, here I was with a doctor who wanted to know what I thought. Who understood that the answer, whatever it was, did not live in the pages of a textbook, or settle at the bottom of a test tube.

So often we think that the truth is a static entity that exists only in a singular place—a place that we have to find. But I have come to realize that the answers I had been looking for, the truth of my own body, was ever-changing. Our bodies have an extraordinary capacity to adapt and survive. Pain is meant to make us pay attention, to warn us, like flares being shot up into the night sky. At first, it's brief: a cry for help that, if it goes unanswered, will only get louder, a flame that, if left unattended, will burn brighter and longer. At first, we find relief in the light because we'd rather fear what it illuminates than what we imagine lives in the dark. We look outside ourselves to explain our pain, because to acknowledge that it is inside of us forces us to recognize it as a part of who we are.

Bodily agonies that do not end beget a kind of forced intimacy with pain that, not unlike other intense relationships, can eventually bleed into something tedious and almost unremarkable in its enduring presence. Its place in our lives can become ordinary and even, at times, oddly reassuring. The moment that pain owns us is not when it chokes our breath, when it knocks us down, or when it steals our pleasure. Pain becomes our master when we wake up one day and realize we no longer fear it. When we come to regard it as not something separate from us, but something of us.

As much as we have labored to resist this in our minds, our bodies acquiesce. Our hearts beat, our cells divide, our nerves—frayed though they may be—fire, and one day we realize that we no longer remember what it feels like to live without pain. What becomes remarkable is not our body's distress call, but the silence. Really, it's the silence that we fear, because it does not mean we have been healed. Silence after pain usually marks our body's inability, or unwillingness, to adapt again, to heal itself, and to persist as we do for an answer, or a reason, for our suffering.

I like puzzles, but I don't like being one. When pain began to court me, I did not care about the why or what-for except for what it meant in terms of getting better. Of being, as I was before, without pain. The only thing that troubled me more than being a mystery was the realization that I was also the one who had to solve it.

As I sat across from Dr. Gish in the exam room, its familiarity neither a comfort nor a concern, I realized that I no longer expected to feel better. I no longer expected to be free from pain. When I first got sick, the motivation to get well was to go back to Sarah Lawrence and resume my life. I believed that the illness was just an interruption, not a complete diversion from the life that I had grown to love so much. I certainly never expected it to change my life, or to become my life. Perhaps I was afraid to believe that it could. I grieved the loss of that life and that vision of myself, but came to marvel at what could fill the emptiness left by the one thing I had been so afraid to lose.

I like to think that it's not that I live in pain, but rather, that I live with it. I no longer feel driven by the need to be liberated from it, or to regain the life it deprived me of. I attempt to identify it rather than identify with it. I tell myself that if I come to understand its intricacies, the mortal magic that bewitches us all in the end, I will strip it of its power over me. The hope of finding the answers, whatever they may be, is a reason to wake up and pull my weary frame from bed. It's a reason to engage in the world around me. I keep looking because I have found answers before. They exist, and I can recognize them. For that, I have proof. I am the proof.

When history and the health-care system obstructed my search, I often took it personally. I felt that I was an unsolvable problem. Through my experiences, I came to realize that it wasn't that the answers didn't exist, it was that medicine, health care, and technology have not coalesced enough to find them. It may be that the answers are not even particularly complicated—but inefficiency, redundancy, and disjunction are adversaries of progress. I know the answers may not help me—but I am not the only one who needs them. That's reason enough to find purpose, and maybe hope, in the search.

But for me, hope's a funny word. Not long before my visit with Dr. Gish, I was on my way home from running an errand a few towns over, idly careening through the back roads, homeward bound. All the snow had melted and the promise of mud was in the air. Farmland had begun to come to life again, anticipating a thaw.

I pulled my car off to the side of the dirt road at the top of a large hill where I often liked to come to feel the weight of my insignificance compared to nature. It looked out over everything—a valley below, the sea in the distance, the hills of the town I called home, and a crisp, wintery blue sky.

No sooner had I settled in did my phone bleep. I picked it up and saw that I had an email from Jane, the subject inquiring. We had had a session scheduled but I was not there—where was I? After being a dutiful patient for almost a decade, rarely, if ever, missing an appointment, and never without calling first, I wasn't surprised that her interest had been piqued.

A series of miscommunications had brought us to this point: we had, in fact, changed the time to be later than our usual appointment, which we had both forgotten. Had I been home, I could have easily driven across town to her office, but as it stood, I was at least fifteen, if not twenty, minutes away. I had taken the long way around the main road and was currently sitting just on the edge of a town called Hope.

I responded to Jane's email, typing, "I would zip over, but I'm on the far side of Hope right now." I meant that I was on the far side of town, but it did strike me as a funny thing to say to one's therapist, and I quickly amended my email to assure her I was not headed for a perfunctory state of hopelessness.

Sitting in Dr. Gish's office some months later, I thought about that phrase: the far side of hope. By then, I was thinking about the emotion, the state of being. I was feeling as though I had come all this way, had waded through so much pain and uncertainty, because I believed I would find the truth—yet here I was, right back where I started. Feeling very much like I was, once again, quite a distance from a hopeful state. The far side of hope, as it were.

CHAPTER 9

Living is a form of not being sure, not knowing what next or
how. The moment you know how, you begin to die a little.
The artist never entirely knows. We guess. We may
be wrong, but we take leap after leap in the dark.

—Agnes De Mille, in *Life*, November 15, 1963

ALTHOUGH DR. GISH HAD DUTIFULLY put in a referral for a neurologist consult, it would be a little over six months before I could get
an appointment. When I called to make it, I repeated my symptoms to
the receptionist, who was presumably setting up a new patient chart
and preparing intake forms. I was a bit anxious about the wait time,
given the nature of my symptoms, and asked her what patients were
usually told to do in the interim. She, of course, couldn't speak for
every patient, but mentioned that her husband had a progressive neurological disease. Her advice to me for the summer? "Use it or lose it."

Of course, my appointment with Dr. Gish had turned up the distinct possibility that I'd already lost it in more ways than one. "It" being a number of things: nerve function, myelin, blood, patience, time,
joy, hope. You can only fail so many neurological exams before you
have to admit that maybe you are lacking some fundamental element
of functioning.

Maybe I was afraid, or bored—more than likely, both—but I decided that when it came to physical functioning, either I could use it

and lose it anyway, or use it and maybe not lose it. So, after seeing a friend's posts about ballroom dance lessons, I took what I hoped would be a proactive leap and signed up for lessons. Ballroom dance, like most styles of dancing—but perhaps even more so, because you have a partner—requires a great deal of physical and mental acuity. Either whatever was going on was going to get worse no matter what I did, or taking some kind of step in the direction of building strength would be fortifying. In other words, I figured it might not help, but it probably wouldn't hurt. More than that, it'd probably be fun—and my life was devoid of many things, but fun had been a concept lost to me far longer than what I could blame on illness. I once looked after a very wise young girl when her mother would go out of town on business, and one evening, she studied me over her dinner and proffered, with the kind of shrewd assessment only preteens are capable of, "You don't have enough fun."

I was somewhat relieved to find that not only were the lessons enjoyable, but my body had not completely forsaken its training. It yearned to stretch through its impediments as I *step-step-together'd* around the studio with my instructor—a comely fellow with a boyish grin that belied the fact that he'd been a professional dancer for more than two decades. He both knew and asked little of me, but what he did do—unequivocally and without question from the start—was regard me as a dancer. And I couldn't help but feel my mouth turning up in a little smile at the thought. Even years ago, when I was in the dance studio for hours a day, to be considered a dancer would have meant something to me. Though I stood there with my neck elongated and feet turned out, my unfamiliar angular body ensconced in ballet-pink tights, diaphanous skirts, and leotards that held me up like a corset once again, there was nothing remarkable about my dancing—except that I was doing it.

It was reassuring to feel a little like a human being again, rather than a spook. I'd started to feel as though my life had become both horrible and fascinating on account of my proximity to the void. A life being lived a mere nudge from the hereafter is interesting to observe. People can't help but stare, and it took me a while to realize they weren't really looking at me. They were looking *past me*, as if they might catch a glimpse of kingdom come, like I was some sort of post-existence looking glass. They were staring at whatever was lurking behind me. Yet I'd never turned around and dared to look it in the eye myself. Maybe I didn't have to see it because I could feel it. The same way I could feel my ballroom teacher's hand on the wing of my shoulder—connection, he called it—signaling me where to go whenever I wasn't oriented in the direction my body should be moving. Whether in death or a rumba, I suppose I was doomed to follow.

As I filled up my days with dancing, writing, and overcompensating for a growing number of infirmities (and more gray hairs than I could reasonably pull out, so I started having my hair dyed on the semi-regular schedule of the reluctantly middle-aged), I thought a lot about my internal concept of time.

In my mind I have always internalized the construct visually as the appropriately seasonally adorned calendar on the wall above the chalkboard in Mrs. Neman's first-grade classroom. It walked from January on the far left of the wall all the way to December on the far right. It was a predictable, pleasant passage of time, with ornate, baby-handed drawings of flowers for spring (an impossibly long stretch that seemed like it would go on forever until summer vacation rolled around). Then the months between June and September would go so fast they seemed to dissipate like water on hot tar. I would stare at that calendar while Mrs. Neman read us *Charlotte's Web*, more fascinated by the passage of time than the moral quandaries of a spider.

Adulthood often felt as though the days moved so quickly that I'd sometimes have to skip a few to catch up. Illness, however, stretched them out such that they ceased to have clear beginnings and ends. As I waited for the next doctor's appointment to arrive, I found myself suddenly quite interested in quantum physics. If only I could devise a way to speed up time. Perhaps the answers were to be found somewhere in the month of November—if I could only get there. Maybe they were hiding behind the finger-feathers of those handprint turkeys.

When the appointment finally arrived, I found myself uncharacteristically inarticulate. It may have been a symptom or sign, but in the moment it felt more like trying to navigate uncharted waters. I'd become very knowledgeable about my endometriosis, about my pelvic organs, and about my gastrointestinal tract (with its little stub

from where my appendix's hit on me had failed years earlier). This
time, I was dealing with a body system I had no proper academic
knowledge of, with a specialist whose specialty I did not understand,
and was still very much in the *getting to know you* phase of what had
become a newly chronic set of symptoms on top of the ones I already
had. The layering effect had quickly become overwhelming, and I
was beginning to wonder if it would even be possible to untangle
the threads. It was a challenge that many of my friends in the autoimmune disease community had warned me of. When you become
chronically ill, you have to adjust to your new baseline. You learn
how to be sick as you are. But no one really prepares you for the possibility that one day, you may have to learn how to be *sicker.*

The neurologist wanted me to have another MRI—one on a specific machine, at a specific hospital, a couple of hours away. This
machine was more powerful than any other MRI machine available
in the state, with a higher Tesla range (a Tesla is a measure of the
machine's magnetic field). I was not opposed to this, so long as I
could get it done sooner rather than later. If I waited until after the
New Year, which was about a month away, my insurance deductible
(which I'd met for the year, blessedly) would reset and I'd be slapped
with yet another bill I couldn't pay. In the seven years since I'd had
my first hospital visit, I'd paid down a few of the associated debts, but
many others had ultimately gone to collections. I have never been in
a position to seek medical treatment without first asking, "How much
will it cost?"

So that's how I found myself driving two hours in a blizzard to
have an MRI. I drove in the 4 p.m. darkness at a venerable crawl, icy
snowflakes hurtling through the void like stars. By the time I reached
the exam room, I was relieved to be able to lay down for a few hours.
MRIs have never bothered me, because I'm not claustrophobic, but
the stress of the trip had worked me up. No sooner had they rolled me
into the machine than my heart began to pound painfully in my ears,
my lungs refusing to take in air.

For reasons that I can't explain but am in no position to question,
at precisely that moment the song "I'm on Fire" by Bruce Springsteen began playing on repeat in my brain. It was so preposterous,
so unexpected, that I couldn't help but nearly laugh. My brain got

stuck on a loop of the final verse, something about a freight train running through your head—which I thought was particularly apt, given the circumstances. I imagined the radiologist reading the scans later, making a note in my chart: *"Diffusion weight images demonstrate no evidence for recent or acute ischemia. The ventricles and sulci are within normal limits. There is an approximately 6-inch valley cut through the middle of her soul."*

For reasons that I have to assume were the result of the chasm between the administrative and clinical facets of health care with which I was once intimately aware, it took a month for me to even get a copy of the MRI report (which turned up no trace of The Boss). Fortunately, they did not find any emergent explanation for my symptoms (a tumor, a lesion, a bleed), but what they did find wasn't exactly normal. The question being, was any of it enough to cause symptoms? And would the symptoms caused match up with the ones I had?

The neurologist had come up with a diagnosis, but I wasn't convinced of it because I didn't really fit the diagnostic criteria. It felt like she was just trying to give me a diagnosis so I'd leave. I hadn't come for a diagnosis, though. Not for the sake of having one, anyway. I only wanted a diagnosis if it was the truth. If there was evidence for it. Proof.

At the same time, I understood that many conditions can only be diagnosed by exclusion—i.e., when everything else is ruled out, it's what's left to explain a set of symptoms. But I'd already seen that episode of *House, M.D.*—you know, the one I'd been living in for over half a decade? All those years of doctors telling me it was "all in my head," or that my illness was "just nerves," seemed to have manifested physiologically: I did have neurological deficits, and I did have demonstrable nerve damage.

My reasons for wanting to understand why were twofold: I wanted to understand why it had happened, so I could either remedy whatever I'd done to cause it, or remedy whatever I had not done to adequately prevent it, and I wanted to know if the cause had any bearing on the other issues I was already dealing with.

I thought a second opinion was reasonable, because taking immune-modulating drugs that one must self-inject is not a decision to be taken lightly. As it was, I was being noncompliant by resisting that intervention despite my doctor's insistence. I didn't need a medical education to be able to look in a neurology textbook and see that I did not meet the clinical diagnostic criteria for the disease she believed that I had, or was destined to develop. Maybe she would be right in the end, but in the meantime, in light of what she was asking me to do, I didn't see why asking for a second opinion was so unreasonable. Of course, as I learned the first time around, referrals were a long process, and I'd already waited six months to see her. The only other test that could, perhaps, provide the kind of proof that I felt I needed was a lumbar puncture, otherwise known as a spinal tap.

A little more than a year after my symptoms first started, and almost six months after my harrowing drive to the Bruce Springsteen MRI, I was curled up like a fetus in her office mulling over the various conditions it could rule in or out (tick-borne illness, infections, multiple sclerosis, cancer) as she stuck a needle between my lumbar vertebrae. As cerebrospinal fluid was tapped out of me like sap from a maple tree, I asked a lot of questions, partly because I was nervous, but certainly also because I was genuinely curious.

I'd always put my faith in science. The health-care system may have failed me at times, and there were certainly limitations of medical research, but the art and science of medicine had often been what saved me. While I recognized that I knew little in comparison to those who had spent decades on an education, my belief in medicine's core virtues persisted irrespective of whether those who were practicing it were doing it well.

When I was home in bed resting, trying to avoid a "spinal headache," which I had been warned was a possibility after the procedure, I marveled for a moment, filled with sudden gratitude that modern science even allowed for such a test to be possible, for it to be safe. How far we had come from James Leonard Corning injecting cocaine into the spines of dogs in his lab and accidentally inventing spinal anesthesia! The very fact that I'd been given a nice dose of lidocaine meant that having a needle stuck in my back didn't feel nearly as bad as it sounded. Whatever discomfort I had felt, during and after, I assumed was par for the course.

I had the tap on the Friday of Memorial Day weekend, which at least meant I'd get an extra day of rest if I needed it. By now my freelance writing career had taken off, and I had quit my job in medical records. I was thankful to be self-employed, because it meant that I could do whatever I needed to do each day to wrangle whatever degree of pelvic pain or nausea—or, as the past year had tacked on, neurological weirdness—was going to plague me. I wrote most of my articles from the bathtub and had, on more than one occasion, muted myself on a conference call so I could retch or have some unexpected bout of diarrhea. I found that physical activity was good for my mind, body, and spirit, which everyone always says—but it was really dancing again that had given me a bit of a lift. It wasn't easy, of course, and it didn't feel like it once had, but I came to terms with that. I was just happy to have something in my life other than pain and work. I had been subsisting on a fairly uninteresting, low-inflammation type of diet, and that worked most of the time. And I had medication for when it did not. I had decided that although my life was quiet, it was not uninteresting. I was grateful to be doing work that I liked, was able to meet and interview and talk to fascinating people all over the world, and looked forward to waking up in the morning to an inbox full of science alerts. I felt so deeply reassured realizing that someone, somewhere, was figuring shit out. Sure, we hadn't figured out how to consistently diagnose, let alone adequately treat, a debilitating condition that had affected millions of women all over the world for centuries—but we finally weighed a dwarf star. Perhaps that sounds a little bitter, and perhaps I was slightly so, but in general I have always been genuinely inspired and grateful for any act of scientific inquiry, regardless of whether it pertained to me. I had always found solace in acts of discovery, no matter how small, and beyond that I simply enjoyed being in awe. My work had gone beyond intellectual passion or even identity: it was hope. Even if I wasn't solving the mysteries of myself or of the universe, I was comforted to know that someone out there was.

About two days after I had the spinal tap, I woke up to my warm, sun-filled bedroom and languished for a moment as my dog, Whimsy, tunneled her way out from under the blankets. My daily routine is about as tedious as it gets: I'm awake by 5 a.m. and working by 6 a.m., though from where depends on how I feel. In fact, the only reason I can work as much as I do is that because most days, I either work from bed, or from the bathtub, or vacillate between the two. It hadn't taken me long to Macgyver something of a workspace so that I could work from the couch as well. If I'm on a conference call, the probability of me being horizontal is very high. If it's after 2 p.m., the chances of me dialing in from the tub are exponentially high. I tended to feel best in those early morning hours, so that's when I went for long walks with Whimsy, made doctor's appointments, or ran errands. I'd work through the morning, make sure Whim got out again sometime around when normal people would be on their lunch hour, and then brace myself for the inevitable misery of the afternoon hours. I almost always required a nap, or if not actual sleep, then a lie-down with a heating pad. But, unlike when I was working in a hospital or an office, being home meant it was possible for me to do that—and that made all the difference.

Invariably, every day started off the same: I took my medication and went pee. So, when I awoke that lazy Sunday morning as I basked in the sunlight, Whimsy's snout pressed to my ear, and realized that I did not feel as though I had to empty my bladder, I frowned. I hadn't had to pee the morning before, either. In fact, I hadn't gone to the bathroom at all in two days. Not only was that unusual, but more than that, I didn't even feel like I had to.

I stared at the ceiling trying to wrack my brain for a rational explanation. I had been catching up on about two years' worth of reading and movies, so more than likely I'd just been so distracted that I'd simply ignored the urge. I was certainly a person capable of being hyper-focused to my own detriment, but, considering how much I'd been instructed to drink to replenish fluids, I would have expected to be about bursting after two full days. Maybe I was dehydrated. Still, it was strange that I *also* hadn't had so much as a twinge in the bowel department: my whole life, I'd tended toward the more frantic end of the irritable bowel spectrum, and I could count on one hand the times in my life when I'd gone more than two days without. Generally, my problem was always the opposite: I was so used to having severe abdominal cramps, even on a relatively normal day of bowel function, that to think I'd gone two whole days with no action—and no consequences of no action—seemed extremely peculiar. I didn't feel bloated or anything—which was another feeling I had become fairly well acquainted with, due to endo's rather extreme version of it.

At that thought, I shot up in bed so fast that Whim actually yipped at the suddenness of it. I threw back the covers and pressed my fingers into the pale, cool flesh of my abdomen, to the basin of my pelvis. I held perfectly still, not even allowing myself to breathe. For the better part of seven years, a dull, heavy ache had taken up residence in the valley of my hip bones. I had learned to tame it somewhat, so it was not always an aggressive pain. But it was always there.

Except now it wasn't.

Whimsy whined next to me and I hushed her, as though I were listening for something, as though that pain was being smothered and if the room was quiet enough I'd be able hear it struggling. But those early morning hours were already quiet. That was why I liked to be up and living in them, when the world was gentler and I could tune in to the frequency of pain that buzzed within me and assess it. Like astronomers listening for extragalactic radio signals or oceanographers listening for undersea seismicity, I had been listening to my body, even if no one else was hearing what I was repeating of its threats. Some days the messages were loud, and I begrudgingly accepted them. Other days my bodily forecast was milder, and those were the days I hoped for most. Whether or not I was pleased by the report, it was always there as long as I tuned in, and I'd learned to live my life by it. Once the shock of realizing that I'd woken up to complete radio silence had subsided, it was replaced by a question that would have been spine-chilling, had I been neurologically capable of detecting that.

Without those dispatches, what the hell was I supposed to navigate by?

WHEN I COULDN'T GET ANY of my doctors on the phone—not altogether surprising, given that it was a holiday weekend—I reluctantly went to the emergency room. Going to the ER always felt like abject failure to me, probably because of all the years I spent working in a hospital hearing how badly patients were shit-talked for doing so (some of which was documented in charts stacked up so high they needed their own shelving unit). Not that I'd been an over-utilizer, or even an incorrect utilizer. I always labored over the decision, and it was only the fact that my symptoms were so bizarre and abrupt that I went. I've always been of the belief that it's what I don't know that will ultimately hurt me, and I don't think it's unreasonable to want to be reassured that the cause of my new symptoms wasn't something serious. Admittedly, I didn't have the slightest idea about what was happening; I was just somewhat stunned by the strangeness of it. And so, too, there was a mounting anxiety, which I certainly hoped would be alleviated by a logical explanation and a practical solution.

This I did not get from the first, nor from the second, trip to the ER that I made in the next twenty-four hour period; nor did I get it from any of the ensuing trips to various doctors over the two weeks that followed. For this, I cannot entirely blame the medical profession. Part of it was my fault—at least in the sense that I had been rendered an ineffective advocate for myself, and I believe that it set the tone for the interactions I had with the health-care system. One of the reasons I quickly became so wearied by the specific predicament I was in was that there could not have been a more potent cosmic nod to what my mother's life had become. What I had always feared *my* life would become if I was not vigilant. After the decades of abuse her body endured, she could no longer have a bowel movement *without* an enema. Although she had stopped vomiting years ago, her days still revolved entirely around what she could eat and the procedure to get rid of it. It broke my heart that even though she had managed to fight back against her desire to purge, her body had eroded such that she still spent so much of her life in the bathroom.

When enemas were prescribed to me, I crawled into my bathroom on my hands and knees so I wouldn't have to see myself in the mirror. I knew what I'd see if I glanced at it: my weight had plummeted firmly into the underweight category since I hadn't been able to eat. Having gone from several regular bowel movements per day to nothing for a week had strangely produced no lower gastrointestinal discomfort, but I certainly felt it referred in my upper GI system. I was still trying to drink as much as possible, realizing that to get any more dehydrated than I already was would just further compound the issue and lock me into a vicious cycle I'd never get out of. To have looked up in that moment and seen a gaunt, dark-haired, sunken-eyed woman in the mirror holding an enema would have been proof of what my racing heart had been asking for days: *Is this going to be my life now, too?*

I had never done an enema before, and since I couldn't feel what I was doing, no amount of Googling was particularly helpful. The bottle emptied, though, so I assumed I'd done it right. As I lay on the floor of my bathroom, I couldn't help but be paralyzed by the feeling that I was seeing the world as Mum did. As she always had. All the years I had been on the outside, never truly privy to what was happening within, but instinctually knowing that I never, ever wanted to be on the other side of the bathroom door. Yet there I was. I tried to rationalize it. I tried to say that it was different, that I was not her, that this was not the same. But as I shivered against the floor, the bones of my hips painfully protruding against the linoleum and my dog scratching at the door—I was stricken by a visceral feeling of failure.

I lay there staring at the ceiling until the alarm on my phone notified me that I had reached the maximum amount of time it was safe to retain the enema—of course, I should have gotten a cramp before that. I had not. In fact, I felt nothing. I yanked myself up onto the toilet and heard the release of fluid and whatever stool had been encouraged by it, but I hadn't felt it. The fact that I'd felt no cramping was disorienting, but at the same time, I was, admittedly, a little thankful. I'd had so much pain over the past few years that even though I was alarmed, I couldn't deny a slight feeling of relief of being pain-free. That feeling was quickly replaced by one of bewilderment and unrest. Not that my situation before had been normal, but over the years it had become *my* normal, my baseline. Such a sudden departure was in and of itself jarring enough, but the fact that the symptoms were so intrusive and cumbersome certainly made it more so. We're taught to be dubious of purported quick fixes, and I thought it went without saying that we ought to be wary of any fixes that just trade one set of problems for another.

When I had attempted to articulate this to the neurologist, she was quite insistent that my need for answers—my "curiosity"—was more than likely what was causing me problems. In her view, I needed a "philosophy" to help me cope—eastern religion or meditation, perhaps, if I was not particularly God-fearing.

I explained how my faith in science had gotten me this far, and that what helped mitigate my anxiety was understanding the problem at hand and forming a plan (or several) for how to deal with it. This approach had, after all, kept me alive for a quarter-century, so I was reasonably confident in it.

"No one is comforted by science alone," she said. She then suggested acupuncture, but I'd tuned out. She sensed as much because then she added, "I know you like to read—"

Ah yes, here we go, I thought. Here comes the accusation.

"—sometimes when you're in medical school you start thinking you have whatever it is you're learning about."

I balked. For nearly a year she had insisted—in the absence of objective evidence, I might add—that I had a degenerative neurological disease. I had been the one who'd resisted, insisting that I didn't fit the clinical profile. That was why I'd agreed to the spinal tap in the first place: it was evidence-gathering—specifically, in the hope that she would not find whatever it was that she was looking for that might lean toward that diagnosis. Which, as it turned out, she did not, and I was glad of it. I certainly hadn't wanted the disease. Frankly I hadn't wanted any disease at all. What I wanted, quite desperately, was for my symptoms to have a comparatively banal and ideally treatable cause. I wasn't there because I wanted a diagnosis for the sake of having one. If I had to have any kind of diagnosis at all, I wanted evidence to support it.

Was this my punishment for questioning her? For demanding evidence before starting a risky, not to mention expensive, treatment? I felt a simmering resentment at her comment that I *liked to read*— meaning, I supposed, that I liked to read up on medical miscellany. The years I'd spent doing so had not been out of interest; I'd been trying to solve a problem. It had been work. If I'd wanted to devote my life to these subjects out of passion, I would have been a biology major, not a dancer. It was only because I had an underlying aptitude for science and a deep respect for the scientific method that medicine as a discipline was something I could assimilate. And after years of working on it, I certainly found aspects of it that I enjoyed. I had to—otherwise it would have been very difficult to stay motivated to forge ahead. But just because I think negative-stranded RNA viruses are fascinating doesn't mean I'm a hypochondriac. Scientists get sick, too, and it's a joke as old as time that doctors make the worst patients. Regardless of my intellectual interests, what my education had given me was a critical eye, a need for replicable proof, and an expectation of thoroughness—and it's my belief that every patient deserves that, whether they have the relevant academic experience to know that they do or not.

One night, about a week into the ordeal, I fell into bed at about six o'clock—which, in early June, was really still daytime. The sun was considering setting and was still quite brightly illuminating my small bedroom. Almost every night of my life I've read before bed, but on this evening I hadn't even the strength to lift the copy of Christian de Duve's *Vital Dust*—which I'd been trying to get around to for weeks—from my bedside table (which was, as a rule, littered with books, tins of Altoids, and several unimpressive succulents). I felt an almost otherworldly pull toward sleep, as though I'd been slipped a sedative or anesthetic. I felt as though every breath I took was particularly shallow, and when I stretched my eyes open, little black holes flickered in front of them like pockmarks on the world around me. Whimsy grunted at my feet, turning her circle on the bedclothes hours earlier than she would have preferred, but seemingly resigned to my unmoving position in bed. The room settled into an uncanny silence that was almost piercing—not to mention next to impossible, given my open window and proximity to a well-traveled street, a quarry, a house with small children, an admirably determined neighborhood skunk, and a lumberyard. The world was then blanketed by pitch-black darkness. I felt drawn in to this alluring void, and at that point I had a very brief but intense and lucid thought: *If I die tonight, what will happen to my dog?*

No sooner had I thought the thought than a complete calm washed over me. There was no tension, no anxiety, no worry—no pain. The last thought I had before I fell into a long night of impenetrable sleep was that if I was going to die, I would die—and there was nothing else I could do about it now.

Besides, Whimsy would be fine. *Dogs survive on instinct*, I thought as I let go.

⸺✣⸺

OBVIOUSLY I DIDN'T DIE, BUT after a few more days of enemas and
no improvement, I did begin to question my life. It may have been
sodium and potassium loss, or just the humiliation of having my own
hand up my ass with such alarming frequency, but by the time my
appointment with Dr. Gish's office rolled around one thing was abun-
dantly clear: I was in no shape to drive.

I had tapped out both Cass and my aunt, who had come to my
aid even when it meant bearing witness to a suppository insertion
in the ER, and since they both worked during the day I didn't want
to trouble them on such short notice for an afternoon appointment.
Hillary, though still my emotional touchstone, was busy taking care
of her rambunctious four-year-old, and Rebecca, while still close to
me in spirit, was living in Brooklyn. The next person who came to
mind was Max's mother, Maggie, who had recently retired. I'd maintained a friendship with her over the years, and as she had a certain
degree of anatomical knowledge herself, I often sought her opinion.
She readily agreed to drive me, and I was relieved. I updated her on
my "condition" as we went to the appointment, but I felt remarkably
tired. She couldn't help but express concern about my weight, and
had it been anyone else I would have bristled. But I knew she wasn't
saying it to be accusatory. She knew it worried me too.

I asked her to come into the exam room with me on the pretense
of needing someone to help me explain what was happening, since I
was so weak that I really wasn't even confident in my ability to speak.
My blood pressure was very low, which explained why I felt so ten-
uously connected to the world around me. The dehydration from the
water loss of several days' worth of enemas couldn't have helped.

Dr. Gish and the nurse practitioner who works with her, Emily,
were perplexed. Although I had been saying I couldn't feel anything
for a week, that had all been subjective, and I knew that. But I didn't
know if there was a way to objectively confirm. Emily said that she
could do a rectovaginal exam, and had I been capable of any kind of
protest I probably would have resisted. I had a long, well-documented
history of painful vaginal exams, and I couldn't imagine that a rectal
exam was much better, even on the best of days. If my brief foray into

a sexual awakening had taught me anything, it was that you didn't jump straight into anal. As I was pondering all this, Emily was looking around the room for the lubricant, which had apparently been pilfered—more than likely by a nurse, but I imagined that, on the list of things that routinely go missing from doctor's offices or hospitals, KY Jelly is probably high up. She excused herself to go look, and Maggie took it as her cue to get up, too—assuming that, while we were friends, we weren't *that* close. Not to mention that my sexual edification had occurred with her son.

She hesitated as she reached the door, regarding me as I sat shaking on the exam table, clutching the crinkly paper dressing to my chest.

"Do you want me to stay?" she asked softly. If she was as embarrassed as I expected her to be, she wasn't showing it. I shook my head, pressing my fisted hands against my chest. So many times over the years I had been in these sterile rooms alone, and I had sought reassurance from whatever was available to me: the perfectly symmetrical organs depicted in diagrams, the untouched test tubes with their limits clearly printed on the side, a bright red box affixed to the wall for sharp and painful things. The doctors may have changed, the years may have changed me, but these items were predictably found in whatever examining room I found myself in. They became totems, touchstones, a trail of breadcrumbs to find my way back through the dark wood, notches to navigate the labyrinth by. A way to spot my turns in this dance, where just when I thought I'd mastered the choreography, the time signature would change.

Maggie had been a dancer, too, and it was with that hard-won, taciturn grace that she glided back into the room. She embraced me without hesitation, as she had many years before. If dancing had made us kindred spirits, we'd remained so because we both understood, without having to explain, that the body had its own vernacular. Many times I've sat in the audience at the New York City Ballet and found myself next to someone who seemed startled to realize they're crying. They always appear to be reacting not just to having been moved, but by the disarming experience of feeling a response, to comprehending something, in the absence of spoken language. Even having danced myself, I am still sometimes taken aback by such occasions: those moments when I hear so clearly something I know only the body can say.

"Wait—did you do it?" I scrambled up from the exam table and looked at Emily as she took off her gloves. She nodded, eyeing me warily. "What the *fuck*," I breathed—reasonably disturbed that I had not felt someone's finger in two orifices of my body wherein you should *most definitely* be able to detect it. I certainly had been able to do so on previous occasions—typically with a great deal of pain.

Dr. Gish and Emily both seemed to think my distress was reasonable, though as they discussed my heightened level of anxiety post-exam, they did not imply that it was causative. It was a sensible reaction—if not one that would invariably exacerbate the situation, which I readily agreed with. In addition to a course of high-dose prednisone (a very strong anti-inflammatory and immunosuppressive medication), they also offered me Ativan, mainly to help me sleep. Especially if the prednisone gave me insomnia, which was one of a laundry list of somewhat intimidating side effects.

Going into the second week of the ordeal, I had to work—even if it meant editing an article on quantum entanglement from my bathroom floor. Not just because I was self-employed and if I didn't work, I didn't earn money—but because I was desperate, once again, to assure myself that my identity outside of any illness was still intact. As I lay curled up on a yoga mat draped with an old towel, I needed work—and the joy and sense of purpose it brought me—more than ever. After a couple of days on the prednisone, I started to feel pain in my back and took it as an encouraging sign that things were "waking up." I still was struggling with the guessing game of when it was time for me to pee, and had reached the point where saline enemas were more of a risk to my electrolytes than they were worth. I tried to start eating solid food again and hoped that my bowel wouldn't obstruct with me unaware.

A few days later, I thought I felt the twinge of having to pee—muted, but present—and I was cautiously optimistic that things would continue to improve. When the course of prednisone finished over the weekend, so, too, did any improvement. Having stopped the steroids and the halting of any progress, I felt quite an emotional comedown, too. I've since learned that's not uncommon coming off steroids, but I think it only stood to increase my pessimism. I relayed these outcomes to Dr. Gish and Emily the following Monday, and they thought it might be worth trying a longer course, tapering the dose over time to mitigate potential side effects and avoid putting my body into some kind of adrenal crisis. Improvement, however slow, was a good sign. Though I remained frustrated and scared, I had quickly adapted to the new routine required of me. Adaptation had always meant survival in my life, and I was not unaccustomed to giving up my preferences, or comfort, or other things lower down on the hierarchy of needs. It was never an easy thing to do, and I harbored significant bitterness about it. But as I let those feelings pass, what was left—in any situation, really—was the simple truth: I could either keep living or die.

Knowing it would likely take several weeks, if not months, to get an appointment, Emily had put in a referral for me to see another neurologist. Even if we were able to resolve the more immediate issue, she and Dr. Gish did agree with me that a second opinion regarding the first neurologist's diagnosis, the one which had led to the spinal tap, was reasonable. Whether or not the spinal tap had anything to do with the current problem became irrelevant as time passed, and I was quickly losing any interest in an explanation. I just wanted to regain normal bladder and bowel function—and, you know, clitoral sensation, which would *come in handy* if people were going to continue to suggest I needed to relax.

As it turned out, the neurologist's office had a cancellation, so he could see me sooner than we'd expected. Emily and Dr. Gish were perfectly happy to get his input on the entire situation, and I allowed myself a particulate of hope. I should not have gone alone, but since it was a last-minute, early-morning appointment—and one out of town—I didn't want to inconvenience anyone. Frankly, I'd started to feel like I was nothing *but* an inconvenience: in the preceding weeks, I'd lost gigs, missed my dance lessons, forgone social events I'd been looking forward to, postponed travel, and, perhaps most gut-wrenching of all, forgotten my best friend's birthday for the first time in twenty years. As I had figured out in the emergency room several weeks before, I no longer seemed capable of advocating for myself. It occurred to me, though, as I sat in the exam room—the ones that never change, no matter where you go, why you're there, or who you see—that perhaps the onus shouldn't have been on me. That perhaps, from where I was, at the mercy of the system, it didn't matter whether I could advocate, because the changes had to come from somewhere higher up.

Dr. Modell was not the first doctor to imply that my symptoms were psychosomatic, but he was the first to literally say the words: "This is all in your head." He also did so in a way that was firmly accusatory, almost to the point of disgust. Especially considering this was not the first time he was meeting me: he had seen me almost ten years before when I'd had that spell of weird leg weakness in high school.

He read through my chart, looked at one of several MRIs that had been done, and before I'd even had the chance to convey that I was *relieved* that he did not think there was a glaring, nefarious process at work, before he even bothered to do a neurological exam, he launched his diatribe. Until that moment, it had not occurred to me to be grateful to the previous physicians who had made these assumptions with, at least, some kindness. While they had been, perhaps, condescending, and at times dismissive, they had not been heartless.

Dr. Modell, however, seemed almost at once repulsed. I felt myself gaping at him, gobsmacked by what felt an awful lot like contempt. When I had arrived, I hadn't been in a very capable place, but the humiliation I felt in his presence rendered me completely defenseless. I stuttered through the conversation, trying to maintain my composure, and was audibly defeated when I finally began to cry. He appeared infuriatingly smug, as though it were all proof to his point. Sensing this, I snapped my head up at him, stealing the air in the room before he had a chance to speak.

"Classic Freudian hysteric, right?" I spat, unsure of who I was more angry at: him, myself, or Sigmund Freud. It wasn't even that he was dismissing me, that he was implying that it was—all of it— psychosomatic, but that he was saying quite plainly that there was no other viable explanation. What angered me, after all the time that had elapsed, was that he was completely invalidating the years of work

I'd done to overcome the trials of my early life. That I, at fifteen years old, had the presence of mind to understand that if I wanted to grow up to be a functioning adult, I needed to begin to work through what had happened to me *as it was still happening.* That at age twenty-six I had lived alone for more years than I had lived with my parents, than I had lived in any kind of home at all. I had struggled through the emotional slog, grieved the loss of the things in life that I had fought the longest for or wanted more than anything. I had taken every antidepressant a doctor asked me to take, every sedative, every mood stabilizer—and all they ever did was make me not care that I felt ill. But never, for one moment of those interventions, did I stop feeling sick.

When I first got sick, I denied it, believing that I ought to be able to will it away. There was no "talking myself out of it," and if the Herculean willpower I'd developed as a child was capable of deferring an illness, it did. That's how I knew when it all began that something had to be truly wrong.

Sitting across from Dr. Modell, with his sour mouth and mocking gaze, I knew that none of that mattered. Only after stating his unequivocal belief did he do a cursory neurological exam—I assumed so that he could document that he did—and I loped through it as my brain tried to process the opprobrium I'd sat through. As he made to reaffirm his stance, I straightened up in my chair and looked at him as calmly as I could. It was clear that he had no intention of ever seeing me again, which was fine by me. All the same, I did have something to say. Even if it was only so that I could hear it.

"Twice before I have been dismissed this way," I said levelly, holding his gaze. He squirmed almost reflexively. "If you look at my chart, it's there."

He hesitated, then sighed, seeming to decide to humor me. "You're clearly very intelligent. Very *clever*," he enunciated. *Bright and wound-tight*, I thought, wincing. I stilled myself, taking in a deep breath before I continued.

"This conversation—both times, this is exactly how it started. I've been here before. Then months, years went by—and I found the answer both times. But by the time anyone listened or took me seriously, these things had gone on long enough to cause damage. To erode my quality of life. I lost years not just to the symptoms, but the search." I exhaled, my shoulders sinking slightly as I became aware of how exhausted I was. "I never wanted to be right," I said firmly, tears making my eyes ache. "I never wanted there to be any-thing wrong. But both times, something was. In this current situation, given those experiences, I don't think it's too difficult to comprehend why I'm attempting to understand what's happening now."

He seemed to consider this a moment, angling himself back in his chair, away from me.

"Well then," he said. "Do you have a theory?"

I swallowed hard. "Not yet," I squeaked. "Before . . . it took a lot of time to research. I'm at the beginning all over again now. I guess . . ." I let my gaze fall, defeated. "I'm just trying to figure out where to start."

"Do me a favor," he said, his voice tinged with the veneer of something destined to become an inside joke. "When you figure out what it is, *let me know.*"

Perhaps I should have taken his *when* as a vote of confidence, but all I heard was the tick of a clock. I wasn't afraid that I wouldn't figure it out.

I was afraid I wouldn't figure it out in time.

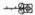

THE GREEK MYTH OF CASSANDRA tells us that she, loved by Apollo, was given by him the power to see into the future. When she rejected him, instead of simply taking away her prophetic gift, he put a most terrible curse on her. Although she could still see what was to come, the curse ensured that no one, not even her own family, would ever believe her when she tried to warn them. Even as her predictions came true—the fall of Troy, the death of Agamemnon—her cred-ibility was eternally doomed. In some versions of the myth, she's imprisoned, because she is believed to have lost her mind—and be-ing locked up actually does drive her insane. Her attempt to escape the fall of Troy ends with her rape by Ajax, and subsequently she is forced to be a concubine to Agamemnon. She even tries to warn him of his wife's affair and his encroaching death at the hands of his wife's lover—which, of course, goes unheeded. Cassandra and

Agamemnon are both murdered by Aegisthus, and, in the end, one wonders if Cassandra had been trying to save Agamemnon after all. For if she'd seen his death, she must've seen her own. In the end, the cruelest consequence of Apollo's curse was that Cassandra couldn't even use her sight to save herself.

EPILOGUE

I BECAME A LEGAL ADULT on June 19, 2007. On June 19, 2017—ten years to the day—I was sweating in a hot bath at six o'clock in the morning, trying to figure out how to end this story. The middling summer heat was already beginning to creep into my apartment. I have perhaps started to outgrow the space—but I am parsimonious, and the rent is very reasonable. The location isn't bad, either: on days when I feel well, I can walk to the waterfront. And my landlord allows me to have Whimsy, my aforementioned mutt, who likes to sit in the doorway to the bathroom. Her birthday—or at least the one I picked for her—was in a few days. The shelter where I adopted her said she was born in mid-June, by their estimate, so I could pick a day if I wanted to. I picked Meryl Streep's birthday. Whimsy will be four in dog years, which, contrary to popular belief, does not equal twenty-eight human years. Though, it would be nice to think we might be at nearly the same place in our respective lives. A cursory Google search explains that she more likely is aging about fifteen years for every one human year she spends with me. I feel as though I have aged at about that rate too. Perhaps that's why my health is what it is: not to say that it's the result of pent-up emotion or unresolved conflict, but rather, an expedited rate of cellular aging in a body that grew up too fast.

The first fifteen years of my life culminated with full, legal adulthood. Ten years later, most of my peers are only just now living on their own. Whether it be getting their first full-time-with-benefits-and-a-retirement-fund job, or querying me about how to get health insurance—since most of them have, up until this year, been covered by their parents' plan under the Affordable Care Act.

As I pruned in the tub, I thought about what I'd hoped, as a teen-ager, my life would be like when I reached this era of it. What I'd hoped my life could become if I made a life-changing—or rather, life-saving—decision. I felt very timeworn at sixteen, and I conflated (as did a lot of other people, I think) exposure with wisdom, and du-rability with maturity. It's only because I realize how young I am right now that I can appreciate how *very* young I was then, and I have a deep and dear respect for that girl.

I know—because I am now and was then a devout list-maker—that I had a clear picture of what I hoped I could achieve if I put the legwork in to fix what needed to be fixed and give myself a solid enough foundation upon which to build the rest of my life. As I had written in my notes-to-self, "I clearly lack some emotional stability and am compulsively analytical, but I'm surprisingly competent and I do hope that counts for something in the end."

Perusing that list—which at the time had seemed like little more than a catalog of fantastic notions—I realized that while I may not have had them all at the same time, there were more things on the list that I had experienced than that I had not. Many of the things I had assumed I would acquire (like an unspecified number of college degrees) were the things that had not worked out, and those which I had deemed to be near-impossibilities (like falling in love with a man who "would tell me I'm interesting or smart instead of just comment-ing on my looks," and "wouldn't be upset if I talked during sex") had manifested beautifully, if only fleetingly.

I studied the list, held it up against the life I have, checking off each wish or aspiration: fulfilling work that I love, living near the sea, having a dog and so many books that I had to start putting the spillover from bookcases in my empty kitchen cabinets. Over the years, I had been able to travel and meet interesting people. My lit-tle brother was happy. I had a few close friends with whom I'd trust my life: I was getting to see Hillary's son grow up and could visit Rebecca at least a few times a year. It was true that some of life's pleasures had been lost to me, and, a bit sadly, soon after I'd discov-ered them: food and sex, mainly. The former may have been the more difficult loss to endure, as I found myself fantasizing about a good pulled pork sandwich more often than sex. I'd been able to dance again, if only for a short time. I even managed to knock some of the more obscure items off the list: that very week, I'd finally acquired an accordion.

As the haves piled up, I began to realize that the one big thing I did not have wasn't even something I'd ever thought to put on the list: my health. Certainly as a teenager it hadn't occurred to me to specifically indicate that I wanted to be in good health—after all, didn't everyone? The closest was my vague sense of not wanting to "end up like Mum," but that worry was laden with a lot more than just concerns of physical health. It had never occurred to me that one day my life would have to be filtered through the sieve of my addled health, thus losing some of its potency each time it passed through the ever-smaller mesh of strain.

Many years ago, Jane scribbled an affirmation on a small piece of paper and handed it to me. I kept it and have it tacked up above my desk: *There is an incredible freedom in letting go of the demand that this moment be anything other than what it is.*

When I was nineteen years old, I woke up one morning and was never the same again. That experience was so jarring and anomalous that I knew exactly what kind of moment it was: a crux upon which my life would always teeter, away from before toward after. There were other moments that revealed themselves more perniciously, the way fledgling autumn nights steal daylight hours and squirrel them away for spring, hoarding light out of the ancient fear of being thrust into the darkness unarmed.

I lift myself from the tub and consider my reflection in the mirror, one that I am strangely relieved to find I do not recognize. It doesn't quite feel like mine, but nor is it my mother's. I often wonder what it is that lived inside her all those years, waiting to take her. I wonder what lived inside of her that kept her alive.

I think of Jane's proffered quote, standing there in my bruised and fragile body with the devil in its details. In that moment, I feel wide awake, wide alive. I wonder what it is that has, for all these years, lived within me, waiting to take me. I wonder what lives inside me now, what's keeping me alive.

It's still early, the day feels mild, and I have work to do. I straighten my spine and turn away from the mirror; I can ask it my questions later. Truth be told, I don't yet know what kind of moment this is. The only thing I know for sure is this: I am in it and I am absurdly alive.

ACKNOWLEDGMENTS

"PRAISE THE BRIDGES THAT CARRIED you over," said Fannie Lou Hamer, and I have always hoped to live up to that. As authors usually indicate, it does take a great many people to write a book. I've also been incredibly fortunate to have a great many people in my life who made living through and eventually reflecting on the events of this book survivable.

I would like to thank my agents, Tisse Takagi and Peter Tallack at The Science Factory, who believed not just in this story, but in me, and my ability to tell it. Tisse provided thoughtful, professional guidance as well as personal support—not to mention amazing tea—and was attentive to the project throughout the process. My wonderful editor, Alessandra Bastagli at Nation Books, immediately understood this book, and therefore me. Her commitment to and belief in this story, her generosity as a human being, and her brilliance as an editor shaped this book and brought it to its full potential. I have learned so much from her and am so grateful to have worked with her. Thanks also to the other members of the team at Nation Books who have championed this book, especially Katy O'Donnell and Jaime Leifer; to my project editor at Hachette, Melissa Veronesi; to Kathy Streckfus for her masterful copyediting, which not only made this a better book, but me a better writer, which is nothing short of a gift; and to Elisa Rivlin for her thoughtful, thorough, and patient legal counsel. And thanks to my publicist Brook Parsons as well, whose guidance has, and continues to be, invaluable.

I would also like to acknowledge the staff of Stanford's Medicine X for giving me a place to share my story, and Susannah Fox and Michael Nielson, who believed it could go further still and set me on the path to get there.

A number of marvelous academics, archivists, and librarians also deserve my thanks, including Heather Pierce-Lopez at Harvard University, those at the Historic Hospital Admission Records Project at Kingston University, and the staff at the Mid-Manhattan Library.

I am grateful to Dr. Tamer Seckin and Padma Lakshmi, Dr. Harry Reich and Liz Reich, and the Endometriosis Foundation of America for giving me yet another space in which to share my story and connect with so many devoted, brilliant minds: Dr. Jay Rosenberg and Lorraine Rosenberg, Dr. Melanie Marin, Noémie Elhadad, and Sylvia English.

Thanks also to the many people at Sarah Lawrence College, from the admissions staff to the friends and professors who changed my life, for permitting me to be part of your community, even for a short while. A degree or thesis could never really capture what I experienced in my time there, and I am forever thankful that I had the chance to thrive. I did so in large part because I had the chance to work with incredible women like Sara Rudner; I hope she knows that I finally learned to let go. I will always deeply admire Elizabeth Johnston for her sharp mind and many achievements and for her kindness and encouragement—not just of my intellect, but of the layers beneath that motivated it.

To some of the many fascinating, loving people in my life:

To Hillary and Jax, to whom this book is dedicated: Hillary, I would not be alive if not for you and that's a fact. If nothing good were ever to happen to me again, my life would still be good and so blessed because you're in it. You are the only person who has been there through every single thing in this book: every couch, every address, every hope and horror, the old pain and the new pain, the old dreams and the new dreams. Perhaps, most of all, thank you for the laughter. There were years where I only laughed with you, and it was not merely life-saving, but life-giving. And Jax, being your aunt is a twofold joy, because from the moment of your arrival I have been able to watch you grow up, and because I've watched your mom become a mother, and that has been such a precious gift to me. I know you're only just learning to read, and while I do hope you'll read this book one day, for now, feel free to stick to *Where the Wild Things Are*.

To Beck: you are a truly remarkable woman, and every year that goes by I find myself feeling luckier and luckier to know you, to call you my friend, my family, really. I'm also incredibly proud of you, and so many times throughout this journey I've wished that I was more like you. I hope you know how much you, and the strength of your convictions, have always inspired me.

To the dear people who have, over the years, loved me in some way, or let me love them: Dagney and Bill; Meg and John; Trish, Kriste, and Alayna; DSK and AK; MPB, BMB, and IPB; DRW, AG, MAM, DCW, Stephanie Cabral, Brett Willard, Sergeant Clapp, Kerry C., Jacob and Julia; Abbie Kopf; and Annika and Rhianna (I'm having a bit more fun now, Rhi—I promise).

I can't even begin to express my gratitude to the woman herein called Jane: "With or without our knowledge, we are all alchemists" (Eric Micha'el Leventhal).

To Liz for taking a chance on me and giving me so many opportunities: I am forever grateful and indebted to you for that, and so thankful to have had your mentorship.

To Stefanie McAllister, for so candidly and fearlessly sharing her story with me: you'll always be the Peter to my Wendy-lady.

To Seth, Jessica, Emma, and AJ: you were kinder to me than I deserved in the very early days of this book's life, and I've not forgotten that.

To the people who may not realize what a vital impact they have had on my life through its many splendid details—the finest of which is coffee, for which I thank Sondra and her Zootlings, Joyce, Richard, and Kathleen Meil, and all the other "townies."

In addition, I would like to thank the following:

The women who have kept the Ask Me About My Uterus community alive online, specifically Rachel C. Charlton-Dailey, Amie Newman, Kara Rota, and Tracey Fischer, who all volunteered their time, expertise, and experiences.

The editorial and creative teams at Futurism, Anchor.fm, Romper, Hippocampus Magazine, Paste Magazine, Medium, and other places I was actively working and writing throughout this process, who provided incredible professional and personal support.

The National Partnership for Women and Families, for giving me opportunities for what's next.

David Streitfeld at the *New York Times*, for mentioning this book before it even had a title, and for the encouraging email exchanges.

Photographer Tim Sullivan of Rockland, Maine, for my author photo.

I couldn't stand the thought of being an ungrateful fangirl, so my thanks to Chris Carter for creating *The X-Files*, and thus, the character of Dana Scully. That being said, I must thank the incomparable Gillian Anderson, without whom Scully would not have become the icon that she is. I used to feel a bit silly about how much a fictional character has meant to me, but I recognize now that in the absence of such a real-life role model during my most formative years, she was an invaluable paragon. I also can't mention *The X-Files* without also expressing my thanks to Anne Simon for her hospitality and mentorship, and, of course, for bringing real science to the show, and thus to me.

Not least of all, I have deep, enduring love and empathy for my parents: you did the best you knew how when presented with a succession of difficult decisions and circumstances that I would think anyone, anywhere, would have struggled to overcome, even in the best of times and with a lot more support.

Thanks also to Nancy and Charles Konarski for loving my brother as if he were your own. And to my brother, who is brilliant, and funny, and kind, and whom I love more than he will ever know.

To the medical professionals in the book and those who are not: you are working in a system that isn't working. It's not working for you and it's not working for your patients. I implore you to ask yourselves if there is something you can do from your vantage point to better advocate for your patients and for your colleagues, to support and encourage one another across disciplines, to get out of the silos in which you operate, to find and foster connections, and to give appreciable weight not just to the science of medicine, but to its art. You may have seen yourself, your words, and your actions or inactions in this book, not necessarily because they were you, but because you see yourself in these conversations, in these hospitals and operating rooms. If you are waiting for a patient to walk into your office and force you to shift your paradigm, don't. The change has to come from you first.

To those in the book's pages whose names and identities have been changed or otherwise obscured, but who no doubt recognize themselves: we're all just hobbling through life, and may we all strive to hobble with more awareness, more compassion, and less fear.

Lastly, to my dog, Whimsy—who is too good for this world, too pure.

NOTES

Chapter 1

5   *In the 1940s, a group of researchers:* James D. Hardy, Harold G. Wolff, and Helen Goodell, "Studies on Pain: Discrimination of Differences in Intensity of a Pain Stimulus as a Basis of a Scale of Pain Intensity," *Journal of Clinical Investigation* 26, no. 6 (1947): 1152–1158.

5   *So that's exactly what they did:* J. D. Hardy, H. G. Wolff, and H. Goodell, "Studies on Pain: A New Method for Measuring Pain Threshold. Observations on Spatial Summation of Pain," *Journal of Clinical Investigation* 19, no. 4 (1940): 649–657.

6   *The results of the study:* J. D. Hardy and C. T. Javert, "Studies on Pain: Measurements of Pain Intensity in Childbirth," *Journal of Clinical Investigation* 28, no. 1 (1949): 153–162.

7   *Of the research that was done:* B. Noble, D. Clark, M. Meldrum, H. ten Have, J. Seymour, M. Winslow, and S. Paz, "The Measurement of Pain, 1945–2000," *Journal of Pain and Symptom Management* 29, no. 1 (2005): 14–21.

9   *Many of my peers:* Patient Protection and Affordable Care Act, 42 U.S.C.§m18001 et seq. (2010) SEC. 2714, Extension of Dependent Coverage.

12   *In June 2005,* Harper's *ran:* Biss's article was titled "The Pain Scale."

Chapter 2

20   *"My ovaries became the center of my universe":* Gilda Radner, *It's Always Something* (New York: Simon and Schuster, 1989).

22   *"Gilda cried," Wilder recalled:* Gene Wilder, "From the PEO-
        PLE Archives: Gene Wilder's Tearful Goodbye to Wife Gilda
        Radner," *People*, posted August 30, 2016, http://people.com
        /movies/gene-wilders-tearful-goodbye-to-wife-gilda-radner, orig-
        inally published in the print edition of *People* in 1991, two years
        after Radner's death.

23   *When I finished reading her memoir:* Gilda Radner, *It's Always
        Something* (New York: Simon and Schuster, 1989), audiobook.

24   *The symbolism was based in:* Edina Gradvohl, "The Toad and
        the Uterus: The Symbolics of Inscribed Frogs," *Sylloge Epigraph-
        ica Barcinonensis*, 2012, www.raco.cat/index.php/SEBarc/article
        /view/264048.

24   *It was all supposedly explained by:* Edward Shorter, *From Paral-
        ysis to Fatigue: A History of Psychosomatic Illness in the Modern
        Era* (New York: Free Press, 1993).

25   *This development came in part:* J. M. Charcot, *Clinical Lectures
        on the Diseases of the Nervous System*, vol. 3 (London: New
        Sydenham Society, 1877), ebook.

26   *They were an integral component:* Jean Martin Charcot, *Lectures
        on the Localisation of Cerebral and Spinal Diseases*, translated
        by Walter Baugh Hadden (London: New Sydenham Society,
        1883).

27   *"If this be a female, and notably selfish . . .":* Susan Wells, *Out
        of the Dead House: Nineteenth-Century Women Physicians and
        the Writing of Medicine* (Madison: University of Wisconsin Press,
        2012).

31   *Humoring me with a more thorough investigation:* Josef Breuer
        and Sigmund Freud, *Studies on Hysteria* (Lexington, KY: Forgot-
        ten Books, 2012).

32   *In 1962, when she was seventeen years old:* Karen Armstrong,
        The Spiral Staircase (New York: Anchor Books, 2005).

41   *I was sitting on the couch at Cass's:* Chris Carter, *The X-Files*,
        Fox, broadcast on WFVX-LD, Bangor, 1993, written by Darin
        Morgan, Glen Morgan, James Wong, Frank Spotnitz, Vince Gilli-
        gan, and Howard Gordon, directed by R. W. Goodwin, Rob Bow-
        man, Kim Manners, and David Nutter. The show ran on the Fox
        network, but for several years in the early 2000s it was syndicated
        to both the Sci Fi Channel and TNT.

43   *Shortly before his retirement in 2012:* David Redwine's talk was
        in 2011 at the foundation's 2nd Annual Scientific and Surgical
        Symposium. It can be viewed in its entirety at Endopaedia, http://
        endopaedia.info/origin39.html.

44   *If you put "endometriosis" into PubMed:* "MEDLINE/PubMed
        Resources Guide," U.S. National Library of Medicine, National
        Institutes of Health, https://www.nlm.nih.gov/bsd/pmresources
        .html.

48   *The theory that uterine tissue:* P. J. van der Linden, "Theories on the Pathogenesis of Endometriosis," *Human Reproduction* 11, Suppl. 3 (1996): 53–65.

50   *Some studies cite an incidence of as little:* A. Kim and G. Adamson, "Endometriosis," Global Library of Women's Medicine, July 2008, http://editorial.glowm.com/?p=glowm.cml /section_view&articleid=11.

50   *Many of these studies obtained their data:* R. D. Kempers, M. B. Dockerty, A. B. Hunt, and R. E. Symmonds, "Significant Postmenopausal Endometriosis," *Surgery, Gynecology & Obstetrics* 111 (1960): 348.

50   *In her speech at the Worldwide Endo March:* Jhumka Gupta, "Endometriosis, Social Pathologies, and Public Health," speech at Worldwide Endo March, Washington, DC, March 19, 2016. The full text of this speech is available on the Endometriosis Foundation of America's website at https://www.endofound.org /endometriosis-social-pathologies-and-public-health.

54   *The fetus had endometriosis:* Mike Schuster and Dhanya A. Mackeen, "Fetal Endometriosis: A Case Report," *Fertility and Sterility* 103, no. 1 (2015): 160–162.

Chapter 3

57   *Sybil—the woman with sixteen personalities:* The miniseries was written by Flora Rheta Schreiber and Stewart Stern and directed by Daniel Petrie for Lorimar Productions, 1976.

57   *It was a name given to her:* Flora Rheta Schreiber, *Sybil* (Chicago: Regnery, 1973).

58   *In her book* Sybil Exposed: Debbie Nathan, *Sybil Exposed: The Extraordinary Story Behind the Famous Multiple Personality Case* (New York: Free Press, 2012).

59   *Another drug commonly given to women:* John A. Sours, "Addiction to Daprisal," *Journal of the American Medical Association* 205, no. 13 (1968): 940.

59   *Practically every adult: Young Frankenstein,* written by Gene Wilder, directed by Mel Brooks, Gruskoff/Venture Films, Crossbow Productions, and Jouer Limited, 1974.

Chapter 4

97   *Harry Harlow, a behaviorist:* Gregory A. Kimble, Norman Garmezy, and Edward Zigler, *Principles of General Psychology* (New York: John Wiley and Sons, 1980).

99   *I remember reading:* Deborah Blum, *Love at Goon Park: Harry Harlow and the Science of Affection* (New York: Basic Books, 2011).

109   *Joseph Campell's archetype:* Joseph Campbell, *The Hero with a Thousand Faces* (Cleveland: World, 1949).

Chapter 5

111   *Even before it had a name:* Cecilia Tasca, Mariangela Rapetti, Mauro Giovanni Carta, and Bianca Fadda, "Women and Hysteria in the History of Mental Health," *Clinical Practice and Epidemiology in Mental Health* 8 (2012): 110–119.

112   *Eighteen case studies:* Sigmund Freud, "The Aetiology of Hysteria," in *The Standard Edition of the Complete Psychological Works of Sigmund Freud*, vol. 3, *(1893–1899): Early Psycho-Analytic Publications* (London: Hogarth Press, 1962), 187–221.

114   *"I would without another thought . . .":* Sigmund Freud and Philip Rieff, *Dora: An Analysis of a Case of Hysteria* (New York: Collier Books, 1993).

123   *True conversion disorder:* "Conversion Disorder," National Organization for Rare Disorders (NORD), https://rarediseases.org/rare-diseases/conversion-disorder.

123   *In fact, some research suggests:* "Somatization Disorder," Harvard Health, www.health.harvard.edu/mind-and-mood/somatization-disorder.

Chapter 6

134   *Take this clinical portrait:* J. D. Martin Jr. and A. E. Hauck, "Endometriosis in the Male," *American Surgeon* 51, no. 7 (1985): 426–430.

134   *Another more recent case involved:* F. I. Jabr and V. Mani, "An Unusual Cause of Abdominal Pain in a Male Patient: Endometriosis," *Avicenna Journal of Medicine* 4, no. 4 (2014): 99–101.

135   *His doctors hypothesized:* Masaharu Fukunaga, "Paratesticular Endometriosis in a Man with a Prolonged Hormonal Therapy for Prostatic Carcinoma," *Pathology—Research and Practice* 208, no. 1 (2012): 59–61.

137   *The study that provided the touted:* Allen J. Wilcox, David Dunson, and Donna Day Baird, "The Timing of the 'Fertile Window' in the Menstrual Cycle: Day Specific Estimates from a Prospective Study," *British Medical Journal* 321, no. 7271 (2000): 1259–1262.

138   *When a woman breastfeeds:* K. I. Kennedy, M. H. Labbok, and P. F. A. Van Look, "Lactational Amenorrhea Method for Family Planning," *International Journal of Gynecology & Obstetrics* 54, no. 1 (1996): 55–57.

139   *"A deep, dark and continuous . . .":* Irvine Loudon, "Deaths in Childbed from the Eighteenth Century to 1935," *Medical History* 30, no. 1 (1986): 1–41.

140   *It might seem like an extremely high number:* Greenberg
        Quinlan Rosner, "Survey Reveals Confusion About Menstru-
        ation Abounds," Association of Reproductive Health Profes-
        sionals, May 22, 2006, www.arhp.org/modules/press/SURVEY
        -REVEALS-CONFUSION-ABOUT-MENSTRUATION
        -ABOUNDS--/15.

141   *Recent research from JAMA:* Y. Tsugawa, A. B. Jena, J. F.
        Figueroa, E. J. Orav, D. M. Blumenthal, and A. K. Jha, "Com-
        parison of Hospital Mortality and Readmission Rates for Medi-
        care Patients Treated by Male vs Female Physicians, *Journal of
        the American Medical Association Internal Medicine* 177, no. 2
        (2017): 206–213.

143   *The National Human Rights Coalition:* Kounteya Sinhai,
        "70% Can't Afford Sanitary Napkins, Reveals Study," *Times
        of India*, January 23, 2011, http://timesofindia.indiatimes.com
        /india/70-cant-afford-sanitary-napkins-reveals-study/articleshow
        /7344998.cms.

144   *A researcher and academic named Sara Read:* Read's article ap-
        peared in *Early Modern Women* 3 (2008): 1–25.

145   *"By all love's soft, yet mighty powers . . .":* John Wilmot Roch-
        ester and David M. Vieth, *The Complete Poems of John Wilmot*
        (New Haven, CT: Yale Nota Bene, 2002).

145   *As the legend goes:* Joshua J. Mark, "Hypatia of Alexandria," An-
        cient History Encyclopedia, September 2, 2009, www.ancient.eu
        /Hypatia_of_Alexandria.

146   *"A review of 1,382 . . .":* G. Bruinvels, R. J. Burden, A. J. Mc-
        Gregor, K. E. Ackerman, M. Dooley, T. Richards, and C. Pedlar,
        "Sport, Exercise and the Menstrual Cycle: Where Is the Research?"
        British Journal of Sports Medicine 51 (2017): 487–488.

147   *A major study showing:* Katherine A. Liu and Natalie A. Dipietro
        Mager, "Women's Involvement in Clinical Trials: Historical Per-
        spective and Future Implications," *Pharmacy Practice* 14, no. 1
        (2016): 708.

147   *Methandrostenolone, for example, also known as Dianabol:*
        D. L. Freed and A. J. Banks, "A Double-Blind Crossover Trial of
        Methandienone (Dianabol, CIBA) in Moderate Dosage on Highly
        Trained Experienced Athletes," *British Journal of Sports Medi-
        cine* 9, no. 2 (1975): 78–81.

166   *Anecdotal evidence suggests:* J. Simons and M. P. Carey, "Prev-
        alence of Sexual Dysfunctions: Results from a Decade of Re-
        search," *Archives of Sexual Behavior* 30, no. 2 (2001): 177–219.

Chapter 7

187   *"He calls me Little Miss Neverwell . . .":* Hilary Mantel, *Giving
        Up the Ghost: A Memoir* (London: Fourth Estate, 2013).

188   *American physician Joe Vincent Meigs:* J. V. Meigs, "Endometri-
        osis: Etiologic Role of Marriage Age and Parity—Conservative
        Treatment," *Obstetrics and Gynecology* 2, no. 1 (1953): 46–53.

188   *"As women have the same physiology . . .":* Kate Seear, *The Mak-
        ings of a Modern Epidemic: Endometriosis, Gender and Politics*
        (Farnham, UK: Ashgate, 2014).

188   *The eugenics vibe:* J. V. Meigs, "Endometriosis—Its Significance,"
        Annals of Surgery 114, no. 5 (1941): 866–874.

189   *"Only a fraction of women affected . . .":* K. R. Mitchell, R. Geary,
        C. A. Graham, J. Datta, K. Wellings, P. Sonnenberg, N. Field, et
        al., "Painful Sex (Dyspareunia) in Women: Prevalence and Asso-
        ciated Factors in a British Population Probability Survey," *British
        Journal of Gynecology*, January 25, 2017.

193   *In her review of literature on endometriosis:* Carolyn Carpan,
        "Representations of Endometriosis in the Popular Press: 'The Ca-
        reer Woman's Disease,'" *Atlantis: Critical Studies in Gender, Cul-
        ture & Social Justice* 27, no. 2 (2003): 32–40.

194   *It was called Dexamyl:* N. Rasmussen, "America's First Amphet-
        amine Epidemic, 1929–1971: A Quantitative and Qualitative Ret-
        rospective with Implications for the Present," *American Journal
        of Public Health* 98, no. 6 (2008): 974–985.

194   *Many women alive today:* Ruth Hubbard, *The Politics of Women's
        Biology* (New Brunswick, NJ: Rutgers University Press, 1990).

196   *this particular framing of endometriosis:* Catherine Kohler Riess-
        man, "Women and Medicalization: A New Perspective," *Social
        Policy* 14 (1983): 3–18.

197   *The most oft-cited study:* Diane E. Hoffmann and Anita J. Tar-
        zian, "The Girl Who Cried Pain: A Bias Against Women in the
        Treatment of Pain," *Journal of Law, Medicine & Ethics* 29 (2001):
        13–27.

214   *It's one of New York City's:* Christopher Gray, "Inside the Union
        Club, Jaws Drop," *New York Times*, February 11, 2007, www
        .nytimes.com/2007/02/11/realestate/11scap.html.

Chapter 9

238   *For reasons that I can't explain:* Bruce Springsteen, "I'm on Fire,"
        on the album *Born in the U.S.A.*, produced by Jon Landau, Chuck
        Plotkin, and Steven Van Zandt, Columbia, 1985.

240   *How far we had come:* Alex Looseley, "Corning and Cocaine: The
        Advent of Spinal Anaesthesia," *Grand Rounds* 9 (2009): L1–L4.

247   *Almost every night of my life:* Christian de Duve, *Vital Dust: Life
        as a Cosmic Imperative* (New York: HarperCollins, 1995).

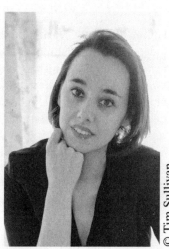
© Tim Sullivan

Abby Norman is a science writer and editor. Her work has been featured in the *Rumpus*, *Independent*, *Paste*, Medium, *Atlas Obscura*, *Seventeen*, *Quartz*, *Cosmopolitan*, and Lady Science/The New Inquiry. As a patient advocate and speaker, she has been on conference faculty at the Endometriosis Association of America, Stanford University's Medicine X conference, and received health literacy training through the Dartmouth Institute. She has been interviewed by *Forbes*, *New York Times*, *Glamour*, *Bustle*, Huffpost Live, and a number of podcasts and international radio programs. She is currently a senior science editor at *Futurism* and the host of *Let Me Google That* on Anchor.fm. She lives on the coast of Maine with her dog, Whimsy.

NATION
BOOKS

The Nation Institute

Founded in 2000, **Nation Books** has become a leading voice in American independent publishing. The imprint's mission is to tell stories that inform and empower just as they inspire or entertain readers. We publish award-winning and bestselling journalists, thought leaders, whistle-blowers, and truthtellers, and we are also committed to seeking out a new generation of emerging writers, particularly voices from under-represented communities and writers from diverse backgrounds. As a publisher with a focused list, we work closely with all our authors to ensure that their books have broad and lasting impact. With each of our books we aim to constructively affect and amplify cultural and political discourse and to engender positive social change.

Nation Books is a project of The Nation Institute, a nonprofit media center established to extend the reach of democratic ideals and strengthen the independent press. The Nation Institute is home to a dynamic range of programs: the award-winning Investigative Fund, which supports groundbreaking investigative journalism; the widely read and syndicated website TomDispatch; journalism fellowships that support and cultivate over twenty-five emerging and high-profile reporters each year; and the Victor S. Navasky Internship Program.

For more information on Nation Books and The Nation Institute, please visit:

www.nationbooks.org
www.nationinstitute.org
www.facebook.com/nationbooks.ny
Twitter: @nationbooks